LESIONS OF THE NERVOUS SYSTEM
IN CANCER PATIENTS

Monograph Series of the European
Organization for Research on Treatment of Cancer
Volume 5

MONOGRAPH SERIES OF THE EUROPEAN ORGANIZATION FOR RESEARCH ON TREATMENT OF CANCER

The Monograph Series of the EORTC deals with selected topics related to cancer treatment. Volumes are usually, but not necessarily, based on the proceedings of an EORTC symposium. The responsibility of the Editorial Advisory Board is to approve the subject of each monograph; the Board does not review individual manuscripts.

Lesions of the Nervous System in Cancer Patients

*Monograph Series of the
European Organization for Research on
Treatment of Cancer
Volume 5*

J. Hildebrand, M.D.
*Head of Neurology
Department of Internal Medicine
Institut Jules Bordet
University of Brussels
Brussels, Belgium*

Raven Press • New York

Raven Press, 1140 Avenue of the Americas, New York, New York 10036

Library of Congress Cataloging in Publication Data

Hildebrand, Jerzy.
    Lesions of the nervous system in cancer patients.

    (Monograph series of the European Organization for Research on Treatment of Cancer ; v. 5)
    Includes index.
    1. Cancer—Complications and sequelae. 2. Neurologic manifestations of general diseases. 3. Metastasis. I. Title. II. Series: European Organization for Research on Treatment of Cancer. Monograph series of the European Organization for Research on Treatment of Cancer ; v. 5.[DNLM: 1. Nervous system—Drug effects. 2. Nervous system diseases—Etiology. 3. Neoplasms—Complications. W1 M0559U v. 5 / WL300 H642L]
RC262.H54   616.9′94′8   78–3000
ISBN 0–89004–269–1

Preface

Approximately one patient in five with generalized cancer will develop major signs of nervous system dysfunction. These complications, which are more likely to occur in advanced stages of the disease, pose a serious threat to the quality and duration of life, and therefore require rapid diagnosis and treatment.

Nervous system disorders occurring in cancer patients can be classified into four broad categories, according to their pathogenesis:

(a) lesions caused by metastases

(b) lesions produced by antineoplastic treatments,

(c) lesions attributed to the remote effect of cancer on the nervous system, and

(d) neurological disorders concomitant with but unrelated to the malignancy.

The purpose of this book is to describe the clinical features, differential diagnoses, and treatment modalities of the first three of the above categories. Presented in the table below is the distribution of neurological abnormalities observed during a 5-year period in 696 patients admitted to the Institut Jules Bordet, Brussels, a general cancer hospital. The data shown indicate that lesions caused by metastases or by local extension of the tumor account for almost 75% of neurological disorders. The pathogenesis should therefore be ruled out first in the differential diagnosis of neurological disorders in patients with malignant tumors. The first three chapters deal with the complications of malignant diseases.

The brain is the most common neural site for secondary localization of malignant cells. The possibility of brain metastases, described in chapter 1, should be considered in any patient with cancer who has local or diffuse signs of cerebral dysfunction. They are particularly frequent in lung and breast carcinomas and in melanomas.

Spinal cord lesions due to metastases are considered in chapter 2. The vast majority of secondary tumors injuring the spinal cord are located in the epidural space, whereas intramedullary metastases are rare.

Metastatic lesions of the peripheral nervous system are described in chapter 3. The spread of neoplastic cells in the leptomeninges (meningeal carcinomatosis) is characterized by the involvement of cranial nerves and spinal roots, together with signs of intracranial hypertension and meningeal irritation. This neurological complication is seen primarily in patients with leukemias or lymphomas and less frequently in those with solid tumors such as digestive, lung, or breast carcinomas. Various clinical deficits may be caused by the compression or infiltration of more distal segments of cranial and pe-

Distribution of neurological disorders in 696 patients with cancer

Nature of lesion	Number of cases	Percent
1. Metastases		
Supra tentorial	206	29.5
Posterior fossa	16	2.3
Cranial nerves	74	10.6
Spinal (intramedullary)	42	6.3
(epidural)	2	
Peripheral nerves (+plexus lesions)	158	22.7
Leptomeninges	12	1.7
	510	73.1
2. Lesions due to antineoplastic treatments		
Surgery	4	0.6
Radiotherapy	5	0.9
Chemotherapy	24	3.4
Infections	10	1.4
	43	6.3
3. Lesions of undetermined etiology		
(Carcinomatous neuropathies)	66	9.5
4. Lesions unrelated to cancer		
Vascular	52	7.4
Toxic or due to carencies	12	1.7
Degenerative + demyelinating diseases	8	1.2
Congenital	2	0.3
	74	10.6

In patients with multifocal or multiple successive neurological disorders only the first diagnosed localization or disorder is reported in this table.

ripheral nerves. Two interesting and common clinical situations in which peripheral nervous system is injured by malignant spread—lesions of the cranial nerves and of the brachial plexus—are also considered in chapter 3.

Lesions of the nervous system caused by antineoplastic treatments occur with less than one-tenth the frequency of metastatic injuries. Their incidence may well increase, however, as the therapeutic approach to the treatment of malignant tumors becomes more aggressive and as new drugs become available for use. The possibility that nervous dysfunctions are due to cancer treatment should be considered in all cases where metastatic lesions have been reasonably ruled out. Lesions attributed to chemotherapeutic drug treatment and irradiations are described in chapters 4 and 5 respectively. Infections of the nervous system, considered in chapter 6, are rare in patients with cancer. They may be regarded mainly, although not exclusively, as a complication of immunosuppressive treatments. Indeed, the responsible infectious agents are similar to those found in immunodepressed patients without neoplastic diseases.

Various pathogenic mechanisms accounting for miscellaneous neurological disorders resulting from vascular and hematological abnormalities are discussed in chapter 7. These disorders are usually attributed to thrombocytopenia, abnormalities of blood coagulation, cardiac lesions, or investigative maneuvers, which favor cerebral embolisms, hemorrhages, or intravascular coagulation. Although none of those disorders is specifically associated with cancer, their incidence is increased in patients with malignant tumors.

A series of so-called carcinomatous neuropathies attributed to a remote effect of cancer on the nervous system are described in chapter 8. Although these diseases were first described 30 years ago, their relationship to the underlying neoplasms remains obscure. In the presence of a neurological disorder in a cancer patient, it is advisable to first eliminate every well-established etiology of neurological disease before considering a still hypothetical remote effect of malignant tumors on the nervous system.

The purpose of this book is to describe the clinical features, differential diagnoses, and treatment modalities of the categories of neurological lesions encountered in cancer patients as noted above. The book will be of interest to neurologists, oncologists, and all physicians involved in the long term care of cancer patients.

Acknowledgments

The author thanks all his colleagues for assistance in the illustration and preparation of this book and Miss Dominique Eeckhoudt for invaluable administrative help.

This work was supported in part by Contract NO1-CM-53840 of the National Cancer Institute, National Institutes of Health, Bethesda, Maryland.

Contents

Foreword

Advances in the treatment of cancer and the progress realized by the use of chemotherapy and other therapeutic methods are creating new problems of patient management because prolongation of life permits the appearance of new manifestations of the disease. Among these, involvement of the nervous system, especially the central nervous system, figures prominently. This was seen most remarkably in acute leukemia, the treatment of which is one of the success stories of clinical cancer research. With the increasing number of remissions and prolongation of the length of remission, leukemic invasion of the central nervous system is seen more and more often and has become a regular feature of the disease instead of a rare complication. This recognition in turn has led to the "prophylactic" or, better expressed, the early treatment of this localization and as a consequence to important new progress in the control of acute leukemia. The same has now been seen with all other forms of tumors, principally cancer of the breast, melanoma, and bronchial carcinoma.

Therefore, progress in therapeutic cancer research makes it mandatory for the oncologist to understand, anticipate, and treat nervous system localizations. That is why a department of neurological oncology has become an indispensable section of a well planned and successful cancer center or cancer hospital. The neurologist-oncologist should be a well trained neurologist in the general sense, but he should also acquire a familiarity with the general aspects of cancer biology and therapy and develop personal experience in the neurological aspects of oncology by seeing and studying the great variety of patients available in the cancer hospital and their neurological complications.

For these reasons, a new branch of oncology requiring extensive training of a multidisciplinary nature has emerged and rapidly established itself. Dr. Hildebrand is particularly well qualified to have written this book, which summarizes in a didactic form the essentials of neurological oncology that everyone needs to know in order to treat patients in a cancer hospital.

Dr. Hildebrand was fully trained in general neurology in the general hospital before becoming a staff member in the service of medicine at the Institut Jules Bordet where he has developed the department of neurology. At the McLean Hospital, in Jordi Folch's laboratory from 1967 to 1969, he also acquired a professional knowledge of the biochemistry of the nervous system. Finally, by association with the experimental chemotherapy laboratory of this Institute, he is fully conversant with the principles and methods of cancer chemotherapy and their special application to a "protected" organ, the central nervous system with its meningeal barrier.

The single authorship of this book explains the well proportioned distribution of the chapters. Even so, the author always speaks from personal experience and from a critical knowledge of the vast literature on the subject.

H. J. Tagnon, M.D.

Chapter 1

Brain Metastases

INCIDENCE AND PATHOLOGY

The brain is the most common site for nervous system metastases of systemic cancers. The proportion of brain metastases compared to other types of brain tumors varies greatly, depending on whether the data are from neurosurgical centers or from unselected autopsy series. Studies summarized in Table 1.1 show that brain metastases usually account for less than 5% of all brain tumors in neurosurgical departments, whereas they account for 37 to 41% in unselected autopsy series. In patients who died from cancer, metastases of the central nervous system (CNS) are found in approximately 10 to 20% (Table 1.1). Authors reporting large series agree that lung and breast carcinoma are the main primary neoplasms in patients with brain metastases (Table 1.2). The primary tumor cannot be identified in approximately 15%. In the vast majority of those cases, brain metastases presumably originate from bronchogenic carcinoma. Indeed, the histology of these tumors is compatible with a pulmonary origin, and it is not uncommon for very small lung cancers to produce brain metastases. In other types of neoplasms, brain metastases usually appear late in the course of the disease, when neoplastic spread becomes clinically evident elsewhere, particularly in the lungs. For instance, the delay between the appearance of the primary tumor and a brain metastasis commonly exceeds 5 years in carcinoma of breast and malignant melanoma (Wilson and Norrell, 1967). Although melanomas account for a relatively small percentage of total brain metastases, it is important to realize that this tumor occurs much less frequently than lung and breast carcinomas. In patients with a generalized melanoma, the likelihood of brain metastases developing is about 50%, whereas the highest corresponding figures reported for lung and breast carcinomas are 40 and 25%, respectively.

There is disagreement among authors about preferential distribution of metastases in certain brain areas (Trevisan and Dettori, 1972). Practically, one may consider that brain metastases are distributed at random, in proportion to the mass of the considered area. Even brainstem metastases, although rare, should not be considered exceptional (Hunter and Rewcastle, 1968; Derby and Guiang, 1975). The most common site for brain metastases appears to be the junction of gray and white matter (Fig. 1.1). This superficial situation makes most of the cerebral metastases accessible to neurosurgical removal. Another very important point before considering neuro-

TABLE 1.1. Frequency of brain metastases

References	Percentage of metastases compared to total brain tumors		Incidence of brain metastases in cancer patients		Type of patients
	No. of cases examined	Brain metastases (%)	No. of cases examined	Brain metastases (%)	
Cushing (1932)	2,023	4.7	—	—	Neurosurgical
Livingston et al. (1948)	1,256	4.1	—	—	Neurosurgical
Christensen (1949)	2,023	3.9	—	—	Neurosurgical
Zülch (1949)	3,000	4	—	—	Neurosurgical
Abrams et al. (1950)	—	—	1,000	17.6	Unselected
Earle (1954)	266	37.2	1,498	11	Unselected
Störtebecker (1954)	4,444	3.5	—	—	Neurosurgical
Simionescu (1960)	195	6.7	—	—	Neurosurgical
Müller and Wochnick (1961)	—	—	3,239	9.8	Unselected
Chason et al. (1963)	—	—	200	18.3	Unselected
Percy et al. (1972)	297	41	—	—	Unselected (including spinal cord)

TABLE 1.2. *Primary tumor site in brain metastases*

References	No. of cases %	Lung %	Upper respiratory tract %	Melanoma %	Breast %	Kidney %	Prostate %	Urinary tract %	Pancreas and gall bladder %	Liver %	G.I. tract %	Reproductive organs %	Endocrine organs %	Lymphomas and sarcomas %	Other %	Undetermined %
Perese (1959)	162	21.6	4.9	7.4	24.1		7.4		1.9		6.2	3.1	3.1	6.2	14.2	0
Brihaye (1963)	184	45.1		4.9	12.0	3.8	0	0.5			6.5	1.6	1.1		6.0	18.5
Richards and McKissock (1963)	389	64.8		1.5	5.9	2.8		0.5	0.3		4.9	0.8		0.3	1.0	17.0
Vieth and Odom (1965)	313	27.5		15.7	16.3		7.0 (+genital tract)				5.1			2.6	11.8	14.0
Paillas et al. (1966)	122	32.8		4.2	17.5	9.2		0.8			9.2	5.0		0.8	3.3	18.3
Hunter and Rewcastle (1968)	393	34.1	1.3	6.1	18.6	9.2	7.3			13.1		4.1	2.5	7.0	0.3	5.6
Order et al. (1968)	108	63.0			13.9	2.8	1.9			0.9	0.9			2.8	6.5	7.4
Nisce et al. (1971)	560	25.0		8.0	39.0										28	
Deutsch et al. (1974)	88	35.2	3.4	5.7	23.9	5.7					4.6	4.6		2.3	2.3	12.0

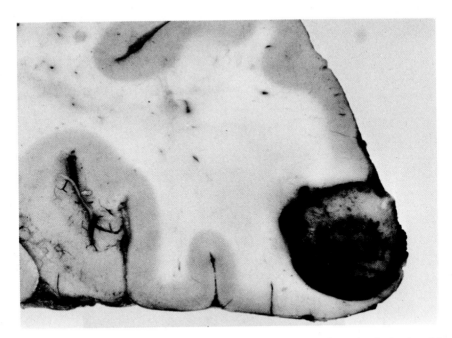

FIG. 1.1. Frontal lobe hemorrhagic metastasis of a bronchogenic carcinoma located at the junction of the gray and white matter. (Courtesy of Dr. J. Flament-Durand.)

surgery is the number of metastases. Here again, as shown in Table 1.3, the figures from neurosurgical centers differ considerably from data from unselected autopsy series. This discrepancy stems from the following: (a) patients seen in neurosurgical departments are selected; (b) their disease is

TABLE 1.3. *Percentage of single brain metastases*

References	No. of cases	Single metastases (%)		Type of study
Livingston et al. (1948)	1,256	72.5		Neurosurgical study
Störtebecker (1954)	125	67	(39*)	At operation (*autopsy study)
Galuzzi and Payne (1956)	741			Bronchogenic cancer only
Ask-Upmark (1956)	696	35.3		Review of literature
Perese (1959)	162	27.8		Autopsy study (includes skull and dura metastases)
Simionescu (1960)	109	56		Neurosurgical study
Chason et al. (1963)	200	14		Autopsy study
Richards and McKissock (1963)	147	26.5		Autopsy study (only bronchogenic carcinoma)
Vieth and Odom (1965)	155	66.5		Neurosurgical study
Deeley and Edwards (1968)	63	47.6		Bronchogenic cancer only, clinical diagnosis
Nisce et al. (1971)	91	60		Autopsy study

not at the terminal stage; and (c) autopsy shows metastases better than any presurgical investigation.

SYMPTOMS AND SIGNS

Approximately 25% of brain metastases are discovered at autopsy. The percentage of asymptomatic brain metastases is particularly high in the pituitary gland. Of 88 cases reviewed by Teeart and Silverman (1975), only six had diabetes insipidus, and one had clinical signs of panhypopituitarism.

All kinds of neurological symptoms and signs may be expected and have indeed been observed in patients with brain metastases; these secondary tumors may be located everywhere in the brain and are multiple in most cases. Therefore, any abnormality of brain function occurring in cancer patients should suggest the possibility of brain metastases.

The most frequent symptoms and signs are summarized in Table 1.4. Early symptoms of brain metastases are polymorphic and are not related to the nature of the primary tumor. Headaches are one of the earliest and most frequent symptoms and respond poorly to analgesics. When they are unilateral, they are located at the side of the tumor in more than 70% of cases (Simionescu, 1960).

Nausea and vomiting are frequently associated with other signs of increased intracranial pressure, such as headache, mainly located in the occipital area, and papilledema. Motor deficits are the most common focal sign. Seizures, consisting mainly of jacksonian attacks, are seen in approximately 20% of patients with brain metastases; they often occur as first signs of the disease.

Paralysis of cranial nerves is often mentioned as a sign of parenchymal brain metastases. The vast majority of cranial nerve lesions, however, in patients with generalized cancer, is due to cranial bone metastases rather than to parenchymal brain lesions. This was the case in 37 of 39 patients with cranial nerve lesions observed by us (see Table 1 in the preface to this volume). The involvement of cranial nerves should also suggest the possibility of carcinomatous meningitis (see Chapter 3) or sequelae of irradiation therapy (see Chapter 5). In rare instances, isolated cranial nerves or their ganglia may be infiltrated by metastases of distant solid tumors (Delaney et al., 1977).

Changes in alertness, intellectual impairment, and gait abnormalities are particularly frequent as first symptoms in unselected populations of cancer patients with brain metastases. Such diffuse signs of CNS involvement heralded brain metastases in 56% of 50 patients observed consecutively in a general cancer hospital (Hildebrand, 1973). The fact that focal lesions are less frequently seen as first signs of brain metastases in cancer hospitals indicates that patients with brain metastases referred to neurosurgeons are highly

TABLE 1.4. Most frequent symptoms and signs of brain metastases

References	No. of Cases	Head-aches (%)	Nausea and vomiting (%)	Motor deficit (%)	Changes of awareness (%)	Aphasia and intellectual impairment (%)	Sensory deficit (%)	Changes of visual fields (%)	Papill-edema (%)	Seizures (%)	Cerebellar signs and/or nystagmus (%)
Chao et al. (1954)	38	55	50	82		53	18		24	21	16
Simionescu (1960)	195	Most frequent symptom (no figures)		36		41			45	29	8
				15[a]		30[a]				25[a]	5[a]
Paillas et al. (1966)	122	61		66		20 (Aphasia)	7	0.8		37	9
		46[a]		16[a]						16[a]	
Order et al. (1968)	108	43		65	8	46	17			26	18
Nisce et al. (1971)	521	33	17	75	41	21	28	15	13	18	19

[a] As initial symptom or sign.

selected and poorly representative of the entire population of patients with secondary brain tumors.

COMPLEMENTARY EXAMINATIONS

EEG, Brain Scans, and Radiological Examinations

Except in rare, refined studies (Rowlan et al., 1974), EEG changes in brain metastases are not considered specific unless multiple lesions are demonstrated. The same is true for isotope brain scan. Both procedures are excellent screening examinations, whereas angiography and computerized axial tomography (CAT) scan are examinations of choice to demonstrate the number and location of brain metastases. In patients with clear-cut focal neurosurgical signs, EEG, isotope brain scan, and angiography demonstrate brain metastases in approximately 90% of cases. However, in patients with diffuse signs of CNS involvement, such as personality changes, alertness impairments, or unsteadiness of gait, these diagnostic procedures (not including CAT scan) show focal lesions in less than 50% (Hildebrand, 1973).

Approximately 40% of cerebral metastases appear on angiography only by displacing normal vessels (Fig. 1.2). In about 50%, neoformed abnormal vascularity may be demonstrated (Fig. 1.3) (Michel et al., 1966). Certain images, named "rims" or "blots" by Trevisan and Dettori (1972), are fairly

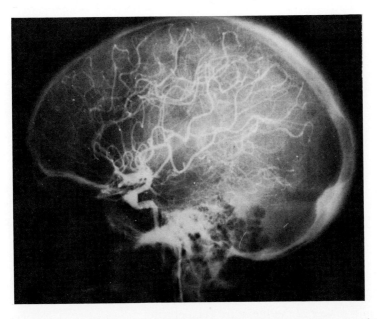

FIG. 1.2. Parietooccipital metastasis of a vascular bronchogenic carcinoma displacing upward the mid-cerebral artery and its branches. (Courtesy of Dr. D. Baleriaux.)

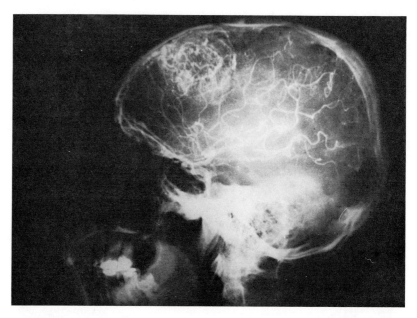

FIG. 1.3. Neovascularization indicating a frontal metastasis of a bronchogenic carcinoma. (Courtesy of Dr. D. Baleriaux.)

typical of brain metastases; other radiological aspects, however, cannot be distinguished from those seen in malignant gliomas or benign meningiomas.

Air studies are hazardous in patients with brain tumors and should be abandoned in the diagnosis of cerebral metastases in centers where CAT scanning is available (Fig. 1.4). This procedure is currently the most accurate method for detecting brain neoplasm (Greitz, 1975) and probably also for assessing tumor growth in response to various treatments. The latter examination will probably gradually reduce the use of angiography in the demonstration of brain metastases (Carella et al., 1976; Norman et al., 1976). It is our belief that at present, angiography should be performed in all cases where neurosurgical treatment is considered.

Cerebrospinal Fluid Examinations

Unless neoplastic cells are found, the analysis of the cerebrospinal fluid (CSF) is of limited help in the diagnosis of brain metastases. Malignant cells are found in approximately 10 to 15% of cases; the highest figure of 30% was reported by Dufresne (1972). Elevation of protein is found in about 50% of patients, but the levels are usually lower than 100 mg/100 ml. Glucose concentrations are normal.

From a review of the literature (Hildebrand and Levin, 1973), determination of enzymatic activities in CSF in patients with neurological diseases ap-

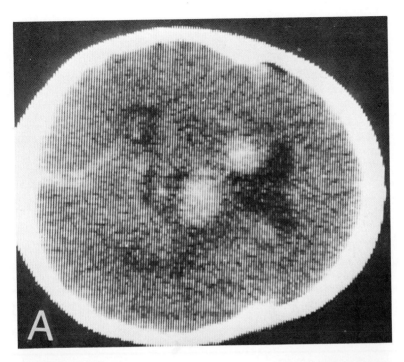

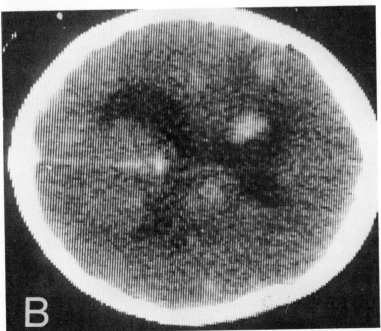

FIG. 1.4. CAT showing multiple melanoma brain metastases at two different levels. (Courtesy of Dr. D. Baleriaux.)

pears to be of limited value. The activity of several enzymes, mainly glutamic oxalacetic transaminase (GOT), lactic dehydrogenase (LDH), and creatinine phosphate kinase (CPK), may be increased in both primary and metastatic brain tumors. These abnormalities, however, are inconstant and nonspecific. Their value is poor, especially in differential diagnosis between tumors and vascular lesions. Determination of phospholipids in the CSF of patients with proven brain metastases was also disappointing in our experience (Hildebrand, 1973). The lack of specificity also limits the clinical use of CSF-plasminogen determination (Kun-yu Wu et al., 1973). The levels of polyamines in CSF have thus far been investigated mainly in primary brain tumors (Morton et al., 1976). Quite recently (Trabucchi et al., 1977), an increase of guanosine monophosphate levels was reported in patients with brain tumors of various origins.

DIFFERENTIAL DIAGNOSIS

Focal Neurological Signs

In patients with an undiscovered systemic neoplasm, the preoperative diagnosis between secondary and primary tumors is almost impossible for space-occupying lesions. In rather rare cases, however, metastases may be identified by angiography. Even when the presence of an extraneural neoplasm is established, the differential diagnosis for such diseases as cerebrovascular lesions or brain abscesses may raise difficult problems. Indeed, in patients with brain metastases, the onset of focal neurological signs is acute in about one-quarter of the cases. Among these, hemiparesis is most commonly seen (Paillas et al., 1966), mimicking a vascular stroke (Hildebrand, 1973). In such patients, complementary examinations could establish the diagnosis of brain metastases by showing multiple focal lesions. Also, if the isotopic brain scan is positive within 24 to 48 hr after the onset of neurological signs, tumors are much more likely than cerebrovascular disease.

The diagnosis of brain metastases may be made even more difficult by spontaneous temporary remissions, which have been observed in 18% of patients by Paillas et al. (1966). Such evolution is often considered to be characteristic of cerebrovascular disease. The development of edema in areas surrounding the tumor may explain the sudden onset of neurological signs in brain metastases, but the complete mechanism is not fully understood.

Another possible cause of sudden neurological deterioration in patients with brain metastases is gross hemorrhage. The exact incidence of this complication is not known. It most often occurs in patients with chorioepithelioma, melanoma, or bronchogenic carcinoma (Mandybur, 1977). Although multiple cerebral lesions in a patient with systemic neoplasm may be considered as good evidence for the presence of brain metastases, they may be seen in brain abscess or embolism secondary to marantic endocarditis, encountered especially during terminal stages in patients with mucoid carcinoma of the digestive tract (Chapter 7).

Other causes of multiple cerebral lesions are brain abscesses, which should be suspected in the presence of infections elsewhere in the body.

Diffuse Neurological Signs

When diffuse signs of CNS involvement are observed, differential diagnosis should be made from several metabolic encephalopathies (which occur with an increased frequency in cancer patients), such as:

(1) *Hypercalcemia,* which may be caused by bone metastases, production of parathormone-like substance, the E series prostaglandins (Seyberth et al., 1975).

(2) *Hypercapnea,* which is frequent in circumstances where brain metastases are most likely to occur, e.g., in primary and metastatic lung neoplasms. In addition, hypercapnea may mimic space-occupying lesions by producing papilledema.

(3) *Hyponatremia* due to an inappropriate secretion of antidiuretic hormone (Schwartz-Barter syndrome).

(4) *Hypernatremia,* by inappropriate tumor secretion of ACTH.

(5) *Hypoglycemia* due to an excessive production of insulin (or insulin-like hormone) and possibly to an increased consumption of glucose by tumor cells.

MANAGEMENT OF CEREBRAL METASTASES

The choice of treatment of brain metastases is determined by three major considerations: (1) their number and location, (2) the nature of the primary tumor, its sensitivity to radio- and chemotherapy, and the extent of the extraneural tumor burden, and (3) the patient's general condition.

Treatment of Peritumor Edema

Steroids are able to improve neurological status, usually within 24 to 48 hr, in at least 80% of patients with brain metastases. The benefit of this symptomatic treatment should be given to all patients with cerebral secondary tumors. Dexamethasone is usually administered with a total daily dosage of 10 to 16 mg, but higher doses may sometimes produce better therapeutic effects. Although a cytotoxic activity of steroids was demonstrated in several neoplasms, it is believed that the clinical effects of steroids in patients with brain tumors are due to their effect on brain edema surrounding the tumor. Indeed, clinical improvement is not related to the nature of the tumor; it occurs rapidly, usually within 24 to 48 hr, and appears to be related to the degree of brain edema. Corticosteroids to a certain degree normalize the blood-brain barrier by an as yet unknown mechanism. The result of their action is a rapid increase of cerebral blood flow in the peritumoral area (Weinstein et al., 1973; Hadjidimos et al., 1973), which occurs before demonstrable changes of vessel position (Capon et al., 1976).

In emergency cases, perfusions of 20% manitol are temporarily effective in reducing brain edema. Glycerol, given at an average daily dose of 1.5 g/kg body weight p.o. in four fractionated doses, is also effective in controlling brain edema and presents a safe alternative to the use of corticosteroids (Bedikian et al., 1977).

Neurosurgery

Surgery is often performed for brain metastases when primary tumors are not apparent and the diagnosis of metastases uncertain. Even when the diagnosis of brain metastases is established, however, their removal may be considered because these lesions often constitute an immediate threat to life. Several studies (Table 1.5) report interesting rates of survival 1 year after craniotomy and mention exceptionally long survivals. Although the benefit of neurosurgery has not been established in controlled studies, it is reasonable to assume that these long survival times are at least partly due to neurosurgery. There are great differences in long-term survival rates from one study to another, however, and marked differences are also observed in mortality rates. Obviously, such variations are related to patient selection. Fortunately, patients with the best chances of prolonged survival also have the lowest operative mortality rate. Although it is not possible to establish rigid eligibility rules for neurosurgery in patients with cerebral metastases, at least

TABLE 1.5. *Results of neurosurgery in the treatment of brain metastases*

References	No. of cases	Survival		Early death (mortality) (%)
		After 1 yr (%)	After 2 yr or more (%)	
Störtebecker (1954)	125	21.6		24.8
Perese (1959)	16		18.8 (At 2 yr)	56.3
Simionescu (1960)	172	2.3	—	38.4
Furlow (1963)	37		16.2 (At 6 yr) + 2.7 (At 7 yr)	5.4
Richards and McKissock (1963)	287	7.7	3.1 (At 2 yr)	68.5 for biopsies 41.8 partial excision 32.2 total excision
Lang and Slater (1964)	208	35	15 (At 3 yr)	
Vieth and Odom (1965)	155	13.5	5 (At 3 yr)	14.8
Raskind et al. (1971)	51	30	8 (At 3 yr)	12

two criteria emerge from all studies: (1) patients must be in good general condition and thus have a minimal extraneural neoplastic burden; and (2) brain metastases must appear unique after a careful clinical investigation and should appear totally removable. Biopsies and partial resections are accompanied by increased rate of early deaths.

Several authors have stressed that better neurosurgical results are obtained in slowly growing tumors, i.e., in patients with long intervals between removal of the primary tumor and development of brain metastases, and that bronchogenic carcinoma metastases are the least favorable cases.

The decision to operate on metastatic brain lesions should be tempered by recent and future progress of radiation and chemotherapy. Therefore, neurosurgery is best undertaken in tumors less sensitive to chemotherapy and irradiation. Neurosurgery may also aim to relieve signs of intracranial hypertension produced by CSF; this procedure is particularly useful in tumors of the posterior fossa.

Radiotherapy

Radiotherapy is a prophylactic treatment in patients with brain metastases, whose aim is to prolong and improve the quality of survival.

The data of Lang and Slater (1964) indicate that untreated patients with brain metastases have a mean survival of 2 months and a median survival of only 1 month. The survival time of patients treated by radiotherapy, reported in studies summarized in Table 1.6, compares favorably with these historic controls. It is important to stress, however, that in addition to the fact that proper controls are lacking in almost all studies summarized in Table 1.6, certain patients had a craniotomy and received chemotherapy and/or steroids in addition to irradiation. Each of those additional treatments may be active per se; for instance, the combination of irradiation of the brain and oral prednisolone offers, according to Horton et al. (1971), only slightly better results in terms of survival and duration of remission than prednisolone alone in the management of cerebral metastases. The same criticism remains valid when the rate of objective relief of neurological signs is considered.

The usual dosage of irradiations for brain metastases varies from 3,000 to 4,500 rads given in 3 to 4½ weeks. More recently, high-dose, rapid courses have been advocated for shorter hospitalization of patients who have a limited life expectancy. It was observed by Posner et al. (1974), however, that the administration of 1,000 rads as a single dose increases the rate of lethal complications as compared to more standard procedures, at least in patients with intracranial hypertension.

In lung small-cell carcinoma, where the survival of patients was substantially prolonged by systemic combination chemotherapy, the risk of brain metastases appeared to increase during the course of treatment. In these patients, so-called prophylactic irradiation of the brain has been proposed

TABLE 1.6. Results of radiotherapy in the treatment of brain metastases

References	No. of evaluable patients	Neurological improvement	Survival	Scheduled radiotherapy	Other treatments
Chao et al. (1954)	38	63%	8.2 mo. in responders 4.6 mo. in nonresponders	3,000 rads	none
Deeley and Edwards (1968)	61	47% "significant palliation"	14% at 1 yr	3,000 rads in 4 wk	7 had neurosurgery
Order et al. (1968)	108	60% (27% at 6 mo., 5% at 1 yr)	mean: 6.3 mo.	2,500–3,000 rads (in over 75%)	26 had neurosurgery
Nisce et al. (1971)	376	80% (mean duration of improvement = 5 mo.)	of the responders: 20% alive at 1 yr 10% alive at 2 yr	3,000–4,000 rads in 4 wk	steroids used
Montana et al. (1972)	62	56%	28% alive at 6 mo. 12% alive at 1 yr	3,000 rads/2 wk to 4,500 rads/4.5 wk	14 had neurosurgery
Deutsch et al. (1974)	88	"the majority improved"	7% alive at 1 yr	3,000–3,500 rads	17 had neurosurgery; steroids used
Newman and Hansen (1974)	45	27% "good response"	median: 3 mo.	more than 4,000 rads	11 had neurosurgery; 29 received steroids
Shehata et al. (1974)	81	35% excellent response 40% fair response 25% no response	mean: 5 mo.	1,000 rads single dose	steroids used

(Hansen, 1973). Recent studies (Tulloh et al., 1977; Jackson et al., 1977) have confirmed that this treatment significantly reduces the rate of brain metastases in patients with small-cell carcinoma but does not prolong their survival.

Radiotherapy is also effective in the treatment of cranial nerve lesions caused by skull metastases.

Chemotherapy

Until now, the role of chemotherapy in the treatment of brain metastases has been modest. The choice of chemotherapeutic agents is related to the extent of systemic neoplastic spread and the pathology of the primary tumor. Thus, in our experience (Hildebrand et al., 1973), breast carcinoma and brain metastases responded much better to the combination of CCNU, vincristine, and methotrexate than the bronchogenic secondaries. This difference between the response of breast and other brain metastases was observed by Pouillart et al. (1976) for the combination of adriamycin, VM-26, and CCNU.

It has been suggested that drugs known to cross the blood-brain barrier should be selected for the treatment of brain metastases. The rationale for preferentially using such drugs is less evident in the treatment of brain metastases than in primary brain tumors. Indeed, primary brain tumors deeply infiltrate normal brain tissue, and the blood-brain barrier may be preserved on their periphery, where the proliferation index is the highest. Metastases do not usually infiltrate normal brain and there is less reason to believe that the blood-brain barrier is still well preserved in metastatic nodules.

REFERENCES

Abrams, H. L., Spiro, R., and Goldstein, N. (1950): Metastases in carcinoma. Analysis in 1,000 autopsied cases. *Cancer,* 3:74–85.

Ask-Upmark, E. (1956): Metastatic tumours of the brain and their localization. *Acta Med. Scand.,* 154:1–9.

Bedikian, A. Y., Valdivieso, M., and Withers, H. R. (1977): Glycerol, a new alternative to dexamethasone in patients receiving brain irradiation. *Abstr. AARC,* p. 50.

Brihaye, J. (1963): Les tumeurs métastatiques du système nerveux central. *Acta Chir. Belg.,* 62:43–59.

Capon, A., Hildebrand, J., Verbist, J., Fruhling, J., and Baleriaux, D. (1976): Changes in regional cerebral blood flows produced by dexamethasone in patients with brain metastases. *Acta Neurol. Belg.,* 76:325–330.

Carella, R. J., Pay, N., Newall, J., Farina, A. T., Kricheff, I. I., and Cooper, J. S. (1976): Computerized (axial) tomography in the serial study of cerebral tumors treated by radiation. A preliminary report. *Cancer,* 37:2719–2728.

Chao, J. H., Phillips, R., and Nickerson, J. J. (1954): Roentgen-ray therapy of cerebral metastases. *Cancer,* 7:682–689.

Chason, J. L., Walker, F. B., and Landers, J. W. (1963): Metastatic carcinoma in the central nervous system and root ganglia. A prospective autopsy study. *Cancer,* 16:781–787.

Christensen, E. (1949): Intracranial carcinomatous metastases in a neurosurgical clinic. *Acta Psychiatr. Scand.,* 24:353–361.

Cushing, H. (1932): *Intracranial Tumours. Notes Upon a Series of Two Thousand Verified Cases with Surgical Mortality. Percentages Pertaining Thereto,* p. 8. Charles C Thomas, Springfield, Ill.

Deeley, T. J., and Edwards, J. M. R. (1968): Radiotherapy in the management of cerebral secondaries from bronchial carcinoma. *Lancet,* i: 1209–1212.

Delaney, P., Khoa, N., and Saini, N. (1977): Isolated trigeminal neuropathy. An unusual complication of carcinoma of the lung. *JAMA,* 237:2522–2523.

Derby, B. M., and Guiang, R. L. (1975): Spectrum of symptomatic brain-stem metastases. *J. Neurol. Neurosurg. Psychiatry,* 38:888–895.

Deutsch, M., Parsons, J. A., and Mercado, R. (1974): Radiotherapy for intracranial metastases. *Cancer,* 34:1607–1611.

Dufresne, J. J. (1972): Cytologie pratique du liquide céphalo-rachidien. In: *Documenta Ciba-Geigy,* pp. 88–91. Ciba-Geigy, Bâle, Switzerland.

Earle, K. M. (1954): Metastatic and primary intracranial tumors of the adult male. *J. Neuropathol. Exp. Neurol.,* 13:448–454.

Furlow, L. T. (1963): Metastatic tumors of the brain. *Clin. Neurosurg.,* 7:63–78.

Galluzzi, S., and Payne, P. M. (1956): Brain metastases from primary bronchial carcinoma: A statistical study of 741 cases. *Br. J. Cancer,* 10:408–414.

Greitz, T. (1975): Computed tomography for diagnosis of intracranial tumors compared with other neuroradiologic procedures. *Acta Radiol. [Suppl.],* 346:14–20.

Hadjidimos, A., Steingass, V., Fischer, F., Reulen, H. J., and Schurmann, K. (1973): The effects of dexamethasone on CBF and cerebral vasomotor response in brain tumors. *Eur. Neurol.,* 10:25–30.

Hansen, H. H. (1973): Should initial treatment of small cell carcinoma include systemic chemotherapy and brain irradiation? *Cancer Chemother. Rep.,* 4:234–241.

Hildebrand, J. (1973): Early diagnosis of brain metastases in an unselected population of cancerous patients. *Eur. J. Cancer,* 9:621–626.

Hildebrand, J., Brihaye, J., Wagenknecht, L., Michel, J., and Kenis, Y. (1973): Combination chemotherapy with 1-(2-chloro-ethyl-3-cyclohexyl-1-nitrosourea) (CCNU), vincristine, and methotrexate in primary and metastatic brain tumors. A preliminary report. *Eur. J. Cancer,* 9:627–634.

Hildebrand, J., and Levin, S. (1973): Enzymatic activities in cerebrospinal fluid in patients with neurological diseases. *Acta Neurol. Belg.,* 73:229–240.

Horton, J., Baxter, D. H., Olson, K. B., and The Eastern Cooperative Oncology Group (1971): The management of metastases to the brain by irradiation and corticosteroids. *Am. J. Roentgenol.,* 111:334–336.

Hunter, K. M. F., and Rewcastle, N. B. (1968): Metastatic neoplasm of the brain stem. *Can. Med. Assoc. J.,* 98:1–7.

Jackson, D. V., Cooper, M. R., Richards, F., II, Ferree, C., Muss, H. B., White, D. R., and Spurr, C. L. (1977): The value of prophylactic cranial irradiation in small cell carcinoma of the lung: A randomized study. *Abstr. ASCO,* p. 319.

Kun-yu Wu, K., Jacobsen, C. D., and Hoak, J. C. (1973): Plasminogen in normal and abnormal human cerebrospinal fluid. *Arch. Neurol.,* 28:64–66.

Lang, E., and Slater, J. (1964): Metastatic brain tumors. Results of surgical and neurological treatment. *Surg. Clin. North Am.,* 44:865–872.

Livingston, K. E., Horrax, G., and Sachs, E., Jr. (1948): Metastatic brain tumors. *Surg. Clin. North Am.,* 28:805–810.

Mandybur, T. I. (1977): Intracranial hemorrhage caused by metastatic tumors. *Neurology (Minneap.),* 27:650–655.

Morton, L. J., Heby, O., Levin, V. A., Lubich, W. P., Crafs, D. C., and Wilson, C. B. (1976): The relationship of polyamines in cerebrospinal fluid to the presence of central nervous system tumors. *Cancer Res.,* 36:973–977.

Michel, D., Dechaume, J. P., and Kofman, J. (1966): Aspects angiographiques des métastases cérébrales. *J. Med. Lyon,* 47:823–829.

Montana, G. S., Meacham, W. F., and Caldwell, W. L. (1972): Brain irradiation for metastatic disease of lung origin. *Cancer,* 29:1477–1480.

Müller, H. R., and Wochnick, G. (1961): Metastatische Hirntumoren. Beitrag zur

Frage ihrer Häufigkeit und zur klinischen Diagnostik. *Internist (Berlin)*, 2:212–223.

Newman, S. J., and Hansen, H. H. (1974): Frequency, diagnosis and treatment of brain metastases in 247 consecutive patients with bronchogenic carcinoma. *Cancer*, 33:492–496.

Nisce, L. Z., Hilaris, B. S., and Chu, F. C. H. (1971): A review of experience with irradiation of brain metastasis. *Am. J. Roentgenol.*, 111:329–333.

Norman, D., Enzmann, D. R., Levin, V. A., Wilson, C. B., and Newton, T. H. (1976): Computed tomography in the evaluation of malignant glioma before and after therapy. *Radiology*, 121:85–88.

Order, S. E., Hellman, S., Vonessen, C. F., and Kligerman, M. M. (1968): Improvement in quality of survival following whole-brain irradiation for brain metastasis. *Radiology*, 91:149–153.

Paillas, J. E., Soulayrol, R., Combalbert, A., Vigouroux, M., Salamon, G., and Lavielle, J. (1966): Etude sur les métastases cérébrales solitaires des cancers viscéraux. *Neurochirurgie*, 12:337–360.

Percy, A. K., Elveback, L. R., Okazaki, H., and Kurland, L. T. (1972): Neoplasms of the central nervous system. *Neurology*, 22:40–48.

Perese, D. M. (1959): Prognosis in metastatic tumors of the brain and the skull: An analysis of 16 operative and 162 autopsied cases. *Cancer*, 12:609–613.

Posner, J. B., Chu, F. C. H., and Nisce, L. Z. (1974): Rapid course radiation therapy of brain metastases. *ASCO Abstr.* (No. 752), pp. 172.

Pouillart, P., Mathe, G., Poisson, M., Buge, A., Huguenin, P., Gautier, H., Morin, P., Hoang Thy, H. T., Lheritier J., and Parrot, R. (1976): Essai de traitement de glioblastomes de l'adulte et des métastases cérébrales par l'association d'adriamycine, de VM 26 et de CCNU. *Nouv. Presse Med.*, 5:1571–1576.

Raskind, R., Weiss, S. R., Manning, O., and Wermuth, R. E. (1971): Survival after surgical incision of single metastatic brain tumors. *Amer. J. Roentgen.*, 3:323–328.

Richards, P., and McKissock, W. (1963): Intracranial metastases. *Br. Med. J.*, 1:15–18.

Rowlan, A. J., Rudolf, N. De M., and Scott, D. F. (1974): EEG prediction of brain metastases. A controlled study with neuropathological confirmation. *J. Neurol. Neurosurg. Psychiatry*, 37:888–893.

Seyberth, H. W., Segre, G. V., Morgan, M. A., Stweetman, B. J., Potts, J. T., Jr., and Oates, J. A. (1975): Prostaglandins as mediators of hypercalcemia associated with certain types of cancer. *N. Engl. J. Med.*, 293:1278–1282.

Shehata, W. M., Hendrickson, F. R., and Hindo, W. A. (1974): Rapid fractionation technique and re-treatment of cerebral metastases by irradiation. *Cancer*, 34:257–261.

Simionescu, M. E. (1960): Metastatic tumors of the brain. A follow-up study of 195 patients with neurosurgical considerations. *J. Neurosurg.*, 17:361–373.

Störtebecker, T. P. (1954): Metastatic tumours of the brain from a neurosurgical point of view (a follow-up study of 158 cases). *J. Neurosurg.*, 11:84–111.

Teeart, R. J., and Silverman, E. M. (1975): Clinicopathologic review of 88 cases of carcinoma metastatic to the pituitary gland. *Cancer*, 36:216–220.

Trabucchi, M., Cerri, C., Spano, P. F., and Kumakura, K. (1977): Guanosine 3'-5'-monophosphate in the CSF of neurosurgical patients. *Arch. Neurol.*, 34:12–13.

Trevisan, C., and Dettori, P. (1972): Diagnostic problems of cerebral metastases. *Neuroradiology*, 3:216–223.

Tulloh, M. E., Maurer, L. H., and Forcier, R. J. (1977): A randomized trial of prophylactic whole brain irradiation in small cell carcinoma of lung. *Abstr. ASCO*, p. 268.

Vieth, R. G., and Odom, G. L. (1965): Intracranial metastases and their neurosurgical treatment. *J. Neurosurg.* 23:375–383.

Weinstein, J. D., Toy, F. J., Jaffe, M. E., and Goldberg, H. I. (1973): The effect of dexamethasone on brain edema in patients with metastatic brain tumors. *Neurology (Minneap.)*, 23:121–129.

Wilson, C. B., and Norrell, H. A., Jr. (1967): Secondary tumors of the brain. *Dis. Nerv. Syst.*, 37:433–440.

Zulch, K. J. (1949): Häufigkeit, Vorzugssitz und Erkrankungsalter bei Hirngeschwülsten. *Zbl. Neurochir.*, 9:115–128.

Chapter 2

Metastases of Extradural Space and Spinal Cord

Although metastases in the epidural space are fairly common, their frequency is difficult to determine because the spinal cord is not systematically examined in large autopsy series and because spinal cord compression will develop in only a limited percentage of patients with metastases of the spine. For instance, in a series of 168 patients with breast carcinoma reported by Lenz and Freid (1931), vertebral metastases occurred in 59% but spinal cord compression in only 8.7%. The frequency of extramedullary metastatic tumors in patients with cancer varies, according to tumor histology, from 1 to 4% for Bansal et al. (1967), and from 1 to 10% in the study of Barron et al. (1959). In our experience, signs of spinal cord compression developed in 1.3% of patients with cancer.

Table 2.1 indicates the pathological distribution of primary tumors which metastasize in the extradural space. This distribution differs from that described for parenchymal metastases of central nervous system (CNS), both cerebral (see Table 1.2) and intramedullary (Table 2.1). Thus the relative percentage of lung carcinoma is constantly lower, usually under 20%. In contrast, the proportion of lymphomas, including Hodgkin disease (Mullins et al., 1971), and sarcomas is substantially higher in epidural metastases as compared with parenchymal secondary tumors.

Intramedullary metastases are rare compared with those at extradural locations, representing 3.4% (6 of 175) of metastatic spinal cord lesions in the study of Edelson et al. (1972). The figures reported by other authors are even lower: 1.6% (2 of 127) for Barron et al. (1959) and 0.8% (1 of 130) for Strong (1962). Clinical features and treatment of extradural and intramedullary metastases are considered separately.

METASTASES OF EXTRADURAL SPACE

Clinical Symptoms and Signs

Spinal cord and extradural space metastases are among the few locations where a relatively small space-occupying lesion may cause major neurological disturbances. With the exception of the rate of onset and the progression of neurological signs and symptoms, which vary considerably, clinical features of extradural metastases are remarkably similar and are not related to the histological type of the primary tumor.

19

TABLE 2.1. *Primary site of extradural space and spinal cord metastases*

References	No. of Cases	Lung %	Upper respiratory tract %	Melanoma %	Breast %	Kidney %	Prostate %	Urinary tract %	Pancreas and gall bladder %	Liver %	G.I. tract %	Reproductive organs %	Endocrine organs %	Lymphomas and sarcomas %	Myeloma %	Other %	Undetermined %
Extradural Space																	
Törmä (1957)	131	13.7			14.5	16	7.6	1.5	0.8		5.3	10				15	214
Perese (1958)	30	6.6	3.3	9.3	10		10	3.3			3.3	10		40.3			10
Barron et al. (1959)	37	29.7			16.2	8	10.8				10.8	2.7		10.8	8	2.7	
Arseni et al. (1959)	231	16.9		0.9	11.7	3.9	6.9	1.3	0.4	3	(Stomach: 5.2) +1.3	(Uterus: 8.6) +5.2	0.9	4.8		11.2	17.8
Botterell and Fitzgerald (1959)	75	2.7		1.3	2.7	4.0	10.7		1.3	—	2.7	1.3	2.7	41.3	16	4.0	9.3
Brice and McKissock (1965)	145	19.3		0.7	8.3	2.1	5.5	0.7			2.1			13.8 (11.0: Primary)	20.7	0.7	26.2
Vieth and Odom (1965)	78	17.9		5.2	19.2	6.4	9.0				7.7			7.7		12.8	14.1
Auld and Buerman (1966)	50	32		16	4	10	16				4 + 2			10	2	4	16
Bansal et al. (1967)	60	25			20	{ 5 (kidney/prostate)					7	5		{ 17 (lymphomas/myeloma)		5	16.0
Edelson et al. (1972)	100	10		1	23	6	4				4	3		29		20	0
Spinal Cord																	
Edelson et al. (1972)	79	46.8		7.6	11.4	5.1					6.3	2.5	3.8	7.6		2.5	6.3

Back pain localized in the area involved by the tumor is the most frequent initial symptom, found in 80 to 90% of patients. Pain may be elicited by vertebral compression, and is usually increased by straining, coughing, or sneezing. Pain is due mainly to compression of nerve roots and, therefore, frequently has a radicular distribution. It may irradiate bilaterally, especially in tumors localized in the thoracic segment. Compression of cervical or lumbosacral roots produces a decrease or disappearance of myotatic reflexes, weakness, and muscle atrophy. Objective sensory changes in territories corresponding to roots injured by the epidural neoplasm are less frequent and occur later, but hyperesthesia is commonly seen.

The delay between the onset of signs of nerve root involvement, including pain, and first symptoms of spinal cord compression varies from a few days to more than 18 months (Törmä, 1957), depending mainly on the site of the tumor and its growth rate. The onset of spinal cord compression may be abrupt. For instance, in the series of 145 patients reported by Brice and McKissock (1965), symptoms of spinal cord involvement appeared within a few hours in 20.7%. Such a rapid progression cannot be caused by an increase of tumor volume and is presumably related to vascular changes. This mechanism may explain why chances of recovery are poor in these cases, as compared with patients with progressive paraplegia, where signs of spinal cord lesion are attributed to the compression of the nervous structures rather than to ischemia. Experimental and clinical observations of Tarlov (1957) indeed indicate that paraplegia caused by gradual cord compression may be reversible.

Despite these variations in the rate of onset and progression, the pattern of neurological abnormalities due to the compression of the spinal cord by an extradural malignant tumor is fairly stereotyped. In slowly progressive cases, limb weakness and gait difficulties appear first. At this stage, myotatic reflexes are brisk, and plantar reflexes are extensor. Weakness is followed by sensory changes; loss of sphincter control develops next. Ultimately, myotatic reflexes are abolished, and paralysis becomes complete and eventually hypotonic. This sequence is attributed to a selective sensitivity of the spinal cord tracts to compression. Lateralization of tumor may be predicted when one lower limb is involved more or before the other, but a typical Brown-Séquard syndrome is rare (Törmä, 1957).

Complementary Examinations

General investigations may occasionally help to discover systemic neoplasms. Erythrocyte sedimentation rate is frequently elevated. In patients with myeloma, serum proteins often show an abnormal electrophoretic pattern. Specifically, neurological investigations essentially consist of (a) plain radiographs, (b) analysis of cerebrospinal fluid (CSF), and (c) myelography.

X-rays

X-rays are abnormal in at least 80% of patients (Brihaye et al., 1959; Barron et al., 1959; Brice and McKissock, 1965; Auld and Buerman, 1966). Loss of definition of vertebral pedicles is the earliest and most frequent sign. Bone destruction, partial collapse of vertebral body, and paravertebral soft tissue proliferation are other, frequently seen, features. Vertebral metastases of breast and prostate carcinoma may appear as osteoplastic areas. Intervertebral discs are usually preserved.

Analysis of CSF

Lumbar puncture frequently demonstrates a blockage of CSF, which is usually xantochromic and almost invariably contains high levels of protein. Dura mater appears to be an efficient barrier against neoplastic spread, and the presence of neoplastic cells in CSF is unusual (Longeval et al., 1975).

Myelography

Myelography performed with lipid-soluble iodinazed oil demonstrates a partial defect or a complete arrest of the dye. The examination is rarely normal in patients with clinical signs of spinal cord compression. Myelography may also be useful to appreciate the effect of treatment and for patients' follow-up. In patients with complete block, a second cisternal injection may be necessary to delimit the extent of neoplastic proliferation. The limit of the contrast medium in the area of epidural metastasis is typically irregular and fringed (Fig. 2.1).

Intrathecal injection of iodinazed oil almost invariably produces a sterile meningitis usually characterized by an increase of CSF cells, predominantly lymphocytes. In some cases, meningeal irritation may produce neck rigidity and fever within 24 to 48 hr following the examination. The retention of the dye in the subdural space has been considered to be a cause of late-developing adhesive arachnoiditis (Bering, 1950). We have never observed such a complication in more than 250 patients who underwent myelography; however, this could be due to the relatively short survival time of patients with generalized neoplasia.

Differential Diagnosis

The differential diagnosis between metastases and the most frequent primary spinal tumors, both malignant and benign, are summarized in Table 2.2. Spinal cord metastases occur most frequently during the fifth and sixth decade, whereas most of the patients with primary tumor are older than 45 (Rogers, 1958).

Intraspinal angiomas are vascular malformations, which usually occur in

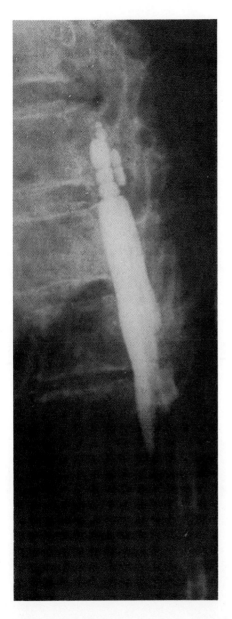

FIG. 2.1. Lateral view of contrast myelography showing irregular and fringed limit of an epidural metastasis. (Courtesy of Dr. D. Baleriaux.)

males under 40 years old; they are mainly located in the thoracolumbar area. Spinal angiography is the most reliable procedure for diagnosis (Aminoff and Logue, 1974).

Meningiomas are found primarily in women, and are most frequently located in the thoracic spine. Pain is less frequent and less intense than in metastatic tumors, and the clinical evolution is slower. Like metastases, neurinomas are evenly distributed along the spine. The clinical features of

TABLE 2.2 Differential diagnosis of main spinal tumors

Diagnosis	Preferential spinal location	Clinical characteristics	Sex age ratio	Average symptom duration	CSF changes	X-ray
Extramedullary metastases	Evenly distributed	Radicular pain invariably present	More frequent in males over 50 yr	Variable; rarely over 1 yr	Protein invariably increased	Vertebral metastases in over 80% of cases; myelography positive.
Intramedullary metastases	Evenly distributed	Pain in 60% of cases, may be radicular	More frequent in males over 50 yr	Within few wk	Protein increased in 80% of cases	Vertebral metastases are rare; myelography normal in 36% of cases
Intraspinal angiomas	Low thoracic Lumbar	Attacks may be followed by symptomless intervals. Pain may cease with position changes	More frequent in males 40–70 yr	2–3 yr	May contain blood	Angiography is choice procedure; tortuous contours on myelography
Meningiomas	Thoracic	Brown-Séquard syndrome more frequent than in metastases; pain less frequent than in metastases	More frequent in women (86%)	2–3 yr	Protein increase is slight	Increase of interpedoncular space; myelography: defect attached to the dura
Neurinomas	Evenly distributed	Symptoms are unilateral, at least at the beginning	No sex predominance; middle-aged adults	3–4 yr	Protein increase is usually marked	Increase of interpedoncular space; enlargement of intervertebral foramen
Gliomas	Most common in cervical spinal cord	Pain less severe than in metastases	Below 40 years old	Over 3 yr	Protein increased	No bone destruction; intramedullary extension on myelography

the two diseases are similar, but their duration in neurinomas is considerably longer and the pain is unilateral, at least during the initial stages of the disease.

Gliomas, along with meningiomas and neurinomas, are the most frequent primary tumors injuring the spinal cord. Unlike meningiomas and neurinomas, they are intramedullary in location. These tumors usually start in young adults; their evolution is slow, compared to metastatic neoplasms.

Symptoms and signs of spinal cord compression may also result from non-tumoral space-occupying lesions, such as extradural hemorrhage or abscess. The former occurs mostly in patients on anticoagulative therapy, the latter in patients with infections, such as osteitis or bacteremia. In patients with purulent collections, symptoms of extradural abscess are acute, but prolonged courses have been observed in cases with epidural granulation tissue (Baker et al., 1975). Prolapse of the intervertebral discs occurs primarily in the lower lumbar segments of the spine and may injure the cauda equina. When based on clinical features, the differential diagnosis with metastases is difficult (Brihaye and Retif, 1969) and may be best established by X-ray examination, which shows collapse of the disc and no vertebral destruction.

Other pathological conditions, such as syphilis, multiple sclerosis, syringomyelia, amyotrophic lateral sclerosis, and combined system degeneration of the spinal cord, may be confused with metastases in patients with generalized neoplasm, although the differential diagnosis is usually rather easy.

More difficult diagnostic problems are raised by postradiation myelopathy (see Chapter 4), especially when a block is shown on myelography, and by arachnoiditis, which may follow the infection of spinal meninges, hemorrhages, or intrathecal injections of various products.

Management of Epidural Metastases

Various treatments of epidural metastases aim for the relief of pain, functional neurological improvement, and increased survival time. Patients' survival, however, cannot be considered as an adequate parameter to test the efficacy of a treatment since it is also related to the evolution of metastases localized elsewhere in the body.

Surgery

Surgical treatment of epidural metastases consists of laminectomy and removal of neoplastic tissue located at posterior and, if possible, lateral aspects of the dura. Laminectomy and biopsy are first indicated whenever a spinal epidural tumor develops as the first event. There is also agreement that laminectomy relieves pain in the majority of patients. It has also been recommended to improve signs of spinal cord compression, despite a high percentage of disappointing results and nonnegligible morbidity and mortality rates (Table 2.3).

TABLE 2.3. Results of treatment of epidural metastases

References	No. of cases	Treatment			Improved	Survival time	Morbidity	Mortality
		Surgery alone	Radiation therapy	Surgery plus radiation				
Wright (1963)	84 { 18 Paraplegic / 47 Paraparetic / 19 Ambulatory	46		38	11%; None became ambulatory / 37% / Not evaluated	Related to tumor type	33% / 47% }	24% (Overall)
Brice and McKissock (1965)	145	136	No details concerning radiotherapy		30% (Overall)	19 patients alive 1 yr after operation	10%	6%
Smith (1965)	52	52	Some received radiation; no details		25% "Significant" / 15% "Minimal"	16 patients alive 1 yr after operation	14%	4%
Vieth and Odom (1965)	78		44	34 (If survival long enough)	38% Not correlated with severity of pre-operative deficit	8 patients alive 1 yr after operation	9%	9%
Bansal et al. (1967)	60	21	9	30	37%	Lung cancer: 41 days / Breast cancer: 5 mo. / Lymphoma and myeloma: 12 mo.	Not given	Not given

Most authors consider as successful results the restoration of gait and sphincter functions; such results have been achieved in about 10 to 35% of patients (Table 2.3). Differences observed in the rate of satisfactory results are related to criteria of patient selection. Thus laminectomy is less likely to be beneficial in patients with abrupt onset of spinal cord compression with severe neurological signs, such as paraplegia (especially when myotatic reflexes are abolished), major sensory loss, and sphincter dysfunction. Patients with primary lung carcinoma are poor responders. There is a certain disagreement concerning the effect of the duration of neurological signs on the outcome of the operation. Thus Brice and McKissock (1965) and Smith (1965) reported higher percentages of favorable responses when symptoms lasted for a longer time, whereas Bansal et al. (1967) made the opposite observation. Surgery should be avoided in patients in poor general condition.

These criteria must not be applied rigidly, for recoveries have been observed even in unfavorable cases. Since best therapeutic results were reported in patients with milder neurological impairment, early diagnosis of epidural space metastases is important. By performing myelographies in patients with radicular symptoms (Mullins et al., 1971) or even with only vertebral metastases (Longeval et al., 1975), the presence of neoplastic tissue in extradural space was detected in at least 25% of patients, allowing early treatment.

Radiotherapy, Chemotherapy, and Hormone Therapy

Radiotherapy when used alone, is effective in relieving pain caused by epidural tumors. It is also given to most patients, after laminectomy, at dosages varying from 2,500 to 3,500 rads. The benefit of irradiation in these patients is based on the analysis of retrospective and uncontrolled studies (Wright, 1963; Bansal et al., 1967).

Chemotherapy may be administered to patients who underwent laminectomy followed by radiotherapy. The choice of chemotherapeutic drugs depends on the histology of the primary tumor and its spread elsewhere in the body. When epidural cord compression is caused by lymphomas, including Hodgkin disease, radiotherapy and chemotherapy may be used without laminectomy (Mullins et al., 1971; Silverberg and Jacobs, 1971), except in cases with rapidly progressive neurological signs. Patients treated only by radiotherapy-chemotherapy combination should be maintained under constant supervision, and laminectomy should be performed if neurological signs fail to improve or become more conspicuous. In patients with lymphomas, the percentage of treatment success is much higher than in those with other neoplasms (Mullins et al., 1971).

Hormone therapy may be used to decrease tumor volume in hormone-dependent neoplasms, such as breast and prostate carcinoma. In addition, the use of corticosteroids has been advised to reduce a possible edema of the spinal cord in patients receiving radiotherapy, especially when laminectomy is omitted. However, the production of edema with the dosages of radiotherapy commonly used in the treatment of epidural metastases has not been established.

INTRAMEDULLARY SPINAL CORD METASTASES

Intramedullary metastases are rare. In 1972, Edelson et al. noted that only 70 cases were reported in the international literature; they analyzed clinical and radiological findings of 29 observations selected from the English literature and in nine of their own patients.

Clinical Signs and Symptoms and Complementary Examinations

When compared with epidural metastases, the clinical picture of intramedullary secondary tumors is less stereotyped. Pain is present in most patients and may be the initial symptom in about one-half of them. Pain may have a radicular irradiation, as in extradural tumors. Weakness is always

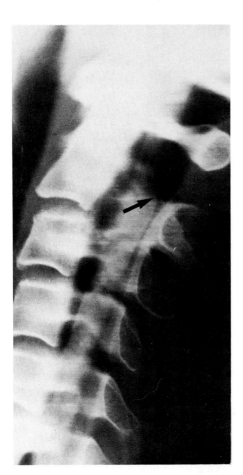

FIG. 2.2. Air myelography showing a widening of the spinal cord, in lateral view (*arrow*) at the level of the second and third cervical vertebrae. (Courtesy of Dr. D. Baleriaux.)

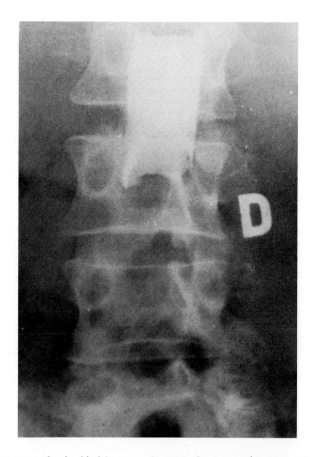

FIG. 2.3. Regular aspect of a dye block in a case of intraspinal metastasis. (Courtesy of Dr. D. Baleriaux.)

present and progresses rapidly; most patients are paraplegic within 2 months. Sphincter difficulties are found in 60% of patients and occur earlier than in extradural tumors. Dissociated sensory loss, considered typical for intra-medullary tumors, is frequent but may be missing (Edelson et al., 1972).

Unlike those seen in extradural metastases, vertebral changes are not fre-quent in intramedullary metastases. In addition, in 30 cases reviewed by Edelson et al. (1972), 13 patients had normal myelography. The most characteristic abnormality found on myelography is a widening of the spinal cord (Fig. 2.2). Its demonstration may require frontal and lateral views. When a complete block of contrast material is present, its limit is more regular than in epidural space (Fig. 2.3). Occasionally, dilated blood vessels are observed above the obstruction on myelography (Edelson et al., 1972) or at operation (Elsberg, 1941). The only frequent change of the CSF is the increase of protein, usually greater than 100 mg%.

The treatment of intramedullary metastases is disappointing. Most patients die or become paraplegic within a few weeks following diagnosis. Laminectomy performed for exploration of spinal cord and biopsy may give temporary relief. It is usually followed by irradiations which are most likely to be effective on lymphoma metastases.

REFERENCES

Aminoff, M. J., and Logue, V. (1974): Clinical features of spinal vascular malformations. *Brain,* 97:197–210.

Arseni, C. N., Simionescu, M. D., and Horwath, L. (1959): Tumors of the spine. *Acta Psychiatr. Scand.,* 34:398–410.

Auld, A. W., and Buerman, A. (1966): Metastatic spinal epidural tumors. An analysis of 50 cases. *Arch. Neurol.,* 15:100–108.

Baker, A. S., Ojermann, R. G., Swartz, M. N., and Richardson, E. P., Jr. (1975): Spinal epidural abscess. *N. Engl. J. Med.,* 293:463–468.

Bansal, S., Brady, L. W., Olsen, A. O., Faust, D. S., Osterholm, J., and Kazem, I. (1967): The treatment of metastatic spinal cord tumors. *JAMA,* 202:686–688.

Barron, K. D., Hirano, A., Araki, S., and Terry, R. D. (1959): Experiences with metastatic neoplasms involving the spinal cord. *Neurology,* 9:91–106.

Bering, E. A., Jr. (1950): Notes on the retention of pantopaque in the subarachnoid space. *Am. J. Surg.,* 80:455–458.

Botterell, E. H., and Fitzgerald, G. W. (1959): Spinal cord compression produced by extradural malignant tumors. Early recognition, treatment and results. *Can. Med. Assoc. J.,* 80:791–796.

Brice, J., and McKissock, W. (1965): Surgical treatment of malignant extradural spinal tumours. *Br. Med. J.,* 1:1341–1344.

Brihaye, J., and Retif, J. (1969): La composante algique monoradiculaire dans les tumeurs de la queue de cheval. *Acta Orthop. Belg.,* 35:679–686.

Brihaye, J., Smets, W., and Derood, M. (1959): Le traitement chirurgical des paraplégies. *Acta Chir. Belg.,* 58:794–810.

Edelson, R. N., Deck, M. D. F., and Posner, J. B. (1972): Intramedullary spinal cord metastases. *Neurology,* 22:1222–1231.

Elsberg, C. A. (1941): *Surgical Diseases of the Spinal Cord, Membranes and Nerve Roots; Symptoms, Diagnosis and Treatment,* pp. 511–512. Paul B. Hoeber, New York.

Lenz, M., and Freid, J. R. (1931): Metastases to the skeleton, brain, spinal cord from cancer of the breast and the effect of radiotherapy. *Ann. Surg.,* 93:278–293.

Longeval, E., Hildebrand, J., and Vollont, G. H. (1975): Early diagnosis of metastases in the epidural space. *Acta Neurochir.,* 31:177–184.

Mullins, G. M., Flynn, J. P. G., El-Mahdi, A. M., McOreen, D., and Owens, A. H., Jr. (1971): Malignant lymphoma of the spinal epidural space. *Ann. Intern. Med.,* 74:416–423.

Perese, D. M. (1958): Treatment of metastatic extradural spinal cord tumors. *Cancer,* 11:214–221.

Rogers, L. (1958): Malignant spinal tumours and the epidural space. *Br. J. Surg.,* 45:416–422.

Silverberg, I. J., and Jacobs, E. M. (1971): Treatment of spinal cord compression in Hodgkin's disease. *Cancer,* 27:308–313.

Smith, R. A. (1965): An evaluation of surgical treatment for spinal cord compression due to metastatic carcinoma. *J. Neurol. Neurosurg. Psychiatry,* 28:152–158.

Strong, R. R. (1962): Metastatic tumour of the cervical spinal cord. *Med. J. Aust.,* 1:205.

Tarlov, I. M. (1957): *Spinal Cord Compression.* Charles C Thomas, Springfield, Ill.

Törmä, T. (1957): Malignant tumors of the spine and the spinal extradural space. A study based on 250 histologically verified cases. *Acta Chir. Scand. [Suppl.],* 225:1–176.

Vieth, R. G., and Odom, G. L. (1965): Extradural spinal metastases and their neurosurgical treatment. *J. Neurosurg.,* 23:501–508.

Wright, R. L. (1963): Malignant tumors of the spinal extradural space. Results of surgical treatment. *Ann. Surg.,* 157:227.

Chapter 3

Meningeal Carcinomatosis and Metastatic Lesions of the Peripheral Nervous System

MENINGEAL CARCINOMATOSIS

Incidence

Meningeal carcinomatosis (MC) is a widespread infiltration of leptomeninges by cancer cells. It occurs more frequently in acute leukemias than in solid tumors. The incidence of MC in children with acute lymphocytic leukemia (ALL) has changed considerably in the last 30 years, first increasing from 5 to more than 50% then falling to less than 5% with the systematic use of central nervous system (CNS)-leukemia prophylaxis.

Before the use of prophylactic treatment, the monthly rate of MC was the same in acute myelogenous leukemia (AML) and ALL: 3.8% during the first 24 months and 2% later (Evans et al., 1970), the higher number of MC observed in patients with ALL being due only to their longer survival. An increased rate of MC is also reported in adult acute leukemia (Dawson et al., 1973) and in the blastic phase of chronic granulocytic leukemia (Schwartz et al., 1975).

The rate of meningeal leukemia (ML) in patients with nonlymphocytic leukemia is even higher when routine cerebrospinal fluid (CSF) examinations are performed in patients in remission, especially elderly ones (Peterson and Bloomfield, 1977). ML is also occasionally reported in chronic lymphocytic leukemia (Amiel and Droz, 1976). The increase of MC rate may be attributed in part to factors such as (a) a better awareness of its signs and symptoms, (b) increased number of lumbar punctures, (c) improved techniques for CSF analysis, and (d) possible immunodepressive effect of systemic chemotherapy. The main factor accounting for the increase of MC in leukemic patients is the prolongation of the lifespan by chemotherapy, which is ineffective against cells present in the subdural space. A similar situation was also observed experimentally in mice inoculated with L1210 leukemia treated with methotrexate (MTX), and in mice with AKR leukemia treated with a combination of amphotericin B plus BCNU: MC was observed only in long-time survivors.

There are no precise data concerning the incidence of MC in patients with solid tumors, but it is likely that the involvement of the leptomeninges by solid tumor metastases is becoming more frequent. Relatively large series of this disease have been reported recently from single institutions (Olson et al., 1974; Little et al., 1974). In Olson's study, 50 cases of MC were collected over a 4-year period, 35 being observed within 14 months. It is also remarkable that MC is now observed in patients with lymphoma, since this complication was formerly rare (Griffin et al., 1971; Olson et al., 1974; Bunn et al., 1976). It is reasonable to attribute this increase of MC rate to the recent progress of chemotherapy in the treatment of lymphomas.

Distribution of Primary Neoplasms

Table 3.1 shows the distribution of solid primary tumors in MC. The most striking difference from tumors that metastasize to the brain and spinal cord is the high percentage of digestive tract neoplasms, particularly of the stomach. The study of Olson et al. (1974) contrasts with other reports by the high percentage of lymphomas and the absence of digestive tumors. Another series of 21 cases of lymphomatous leptomeningitis has been encountered over a 6-year period by Griffin et al. (1971); 15 of their patients had a histiocytic lymphoma. In the study of Bunn et al. (1976), there was also a prevalence of histiocytic and undifferentiated lymphomas in MC due to this neoplasm.

Pathology

In some cases, the gross aspect of the brain may be normal; in others, the leptomeninges are thickened and cloudy. A certain degree of ventricular dilatation may be present. Cranial nerves and spinal roots may be surrounded by neoplastic tissue and appear enlarged or matted together by fibrous tissue, particularly at the level of the cauda equina (Fig. 3.1).

Microscopically, pure leptomeningeal forms of MC are characterized by a diffuse infiltration of the pia mater and the arachnoid by tumor cells (Fig. 3.2). This infiltration usually invades the perivascular spaces of Virchow-Robin and the periradicular sleeves of spinal roots (Fig. 3.3). In addition to the diffuse neoplastic infiltration, nodular metastases of variable size may be found in the meninges and along the spinal roots.

Neoplastic cells may also be present in the cerebral parenchyma, where they are surrounded by a glial reaction. Disappearance of neurons, particularly of Purkinje cells, has been observed. Degeneration of the spinal roots and the cranial nerves, especially the optic nerve, has been reported.

Tumor cells may reach the brain tissue from leptomeninges through the pia or perivascular spaces. In cases where large metastatic nodules are found in brain parenchyma, however, it is believed that MC is secondary to the blood-borne cerebral metastases. Other modes of leptomeningeal invasion have also been considered. For example, Grain and Karr (1955) supported the idea of the meningeal invasion through perineural lymphatics.

TABLE 3.1. *Primary site of solid tumors in MC*

References	No. of cases	Digestive tract (stomach only) (%)	Lung (%)	Breast (%)	Lymphomas (%)	Skin (%)	Other (%)	Unknown (%)
Löwenthal, quoted by Danis and Brihaye-van Geertruyden (1952)	55	34.2 (23.4)	23.4	21.6	—	1.8	18	—
Brucher and Cervós-Navarro (1960) Review of literature 1951–1960	48	43 (33)	33	6	0	0	4	13
Personal cases	11	64 (45)	27	0	0	0	0	9
Olson et al. (1974)	50	0	16	36	28	0	18	2
Little et al. (1974)	29	17 (14)	24	31	0	14	7	7

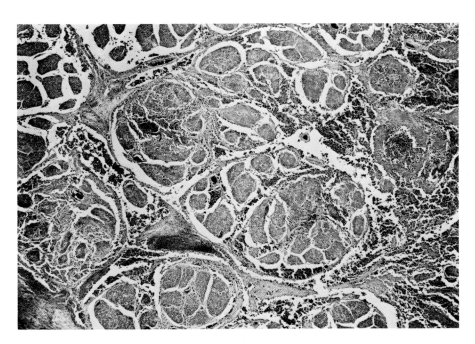

FIG. 3.1. Cauda equina infiltration by a bronchogenic carcinoma. Spinal roots are matted together by neoplastic and fibrous tissue. (Courtesy, Dr. J. Flament-Durand.)

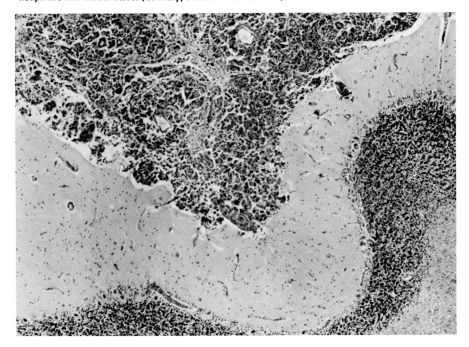

FIG. 3.2. MC due to a bronchogenic carcinoma. The leptomeninges are massively invaded by neoplastic cells. (Courtesy, Dr. J. Flament-Durand.)

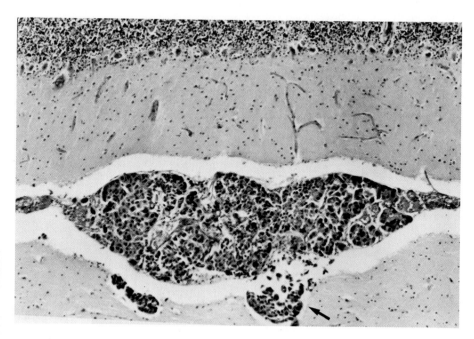

FIG. 3.3. Invasion of a perivascular space (arrow) by neoplastic cells in a MC produced by a bronchogenic carcinoma. ×22. (Courtesy, Dr. J. Flament-Durand.)

Symptoms and Signs

The main characteristic of clinical presentation of MC is the widespread, multifocal, often asymmetrical involvement of the nervous system consisting essentially of (a) encephalopathy and intracranial hypertension, (b) meningeal irritation, (c) cranial nerve lesions, and (d) spinal neuropathy (Table 3.2). The onset of MC is usually gradual and insidious.

Signs and symptoms of encephalopathy or of intracranial hypertension, such as mental changes, confusion, irritability, lethargy, diffuse headache, nausea and vomiting, and papilledema, are the most prominent first manifestations of MC. Although these clinical features are eventually observed in almost all patients who do not respond to treatment, purely spinal forms of MC have been reported (Ardichvili et al., 1971; Parsons, 1972). Signs of focal brain lesions are not frequent; with the exception of the study by Olson et al. (1974), seizures are considered rare. Hyperphagia with excessive weight gain and diabetes insipidus have been reported in about 7% (Pochedly, 1975) of leukemic children. These syndromes are due to leukemic infiltration of the hypothalamus or posterior pituitary gland. Nuchal rigidity is frequently seen, but may be missing at the initial stages of the disease.

Involvement of the cranial nerves is present in the majority of patients with

TABLE 3.2. *Main symptoms and signs of MC*

Type of primary tumor	Acute leukemias (%)	Lym- phomas (%)	Lymphomas and other solid tumors (%)	Solid tumors other than lymphomas (%)		
	Pochedly (1975) adopted from Kanner et al.	Griffin et al. (1971)	Olson et al. (1974)	Grain and Karr (1955)	Brucher and Cervós– Navarro (1960)	Little et al. (1974)
No. of cases	656	18	14 lymphomas 36 other	75	11	29
Encephalopathy				84	73	
Mental and con- sciousness changes	4.7		32			45
Seizures	3.8		26			
Intracranial hyper- tension		44				
Headache	54		50	61	55	59
Nausea and vomiting	54		36	33	36	
Papilledema	50		18	28		21
Meningeal irritation				93	45	48
Nuchal rigidity			34	≤40		
Cranial nerve lesions	9.5 (+visual dist: 5.3)	61	94	68	73	72
Spinal nerve lesions	6.0	39	94 (weakness of extrem- ities)	49	64	
Upper limbs						45
Lower limbs						66
Cauda esquina						21
Other	14.6 (hypothala- mic hyper- phagia in 7.3%)	22 (17% cord compres- sion)				

MC secondary to solid tumors. It is less frequent in leukemic patients than in patients with solid tumors (Table 3.2). The most commonly involved cranial nerves are the oculomotor (III, IV, and VI), facial (VII), and ophthalmic (II) pairs. Blindness may be a dramatic initial feature of MC; it usually appears gradually, but in certain cases the onset may occur within 24 to 48 hr (Danis and Brihaye-van Geertruyden, 1952; Fischer-Williams et al., 1955; Altrocchi and Eckman, 1973).

Like the cranial nerves, the spinal roots are also more frequently injured in solid tumors than in leukemic meningitis. The symptoms and signs of spinal root involvement are radicular pain, stiff back, depression of tendon reflexes, weakness, muscle atrophy, and, less commonly seen, objective sensory changes. Fasciculations were observed in 4 of 13 patients with spinal MC reviewed by Parsons (1972). The deficits due to spinal root lesions are widespread and usually asymmetrical.

CSF Changes

Lumbar puncture is the most useful diagnostic test in MC. Other examinations, such as EEG, brain scan, and pneumoencephalography, may be abnormal but do not contribute to establishment of the diagnosis. Myelography may demonstrate occasional nodular thickening of nerve roots.

In patients with acute leukemia, the diagnosis of MC can be made, even in the absence of clinical signs and symptoms of the disease, when two or more blasts are found in CSF. The use of the centrifuge in the analysis of CSF increased the rate of diagnosis of MC (Evans et al., 1974). Complete disappearance of blasts from the CSF correlates well with clinical improvement, but Aaronson et al. (1975) failed to discover any correlation between the number of blasts in CSF and clinical signs or extent of involvement at pathological examination. In patients with solid tumors, unlike in those with acute leukemia, the presence of neoplastic cells cannot be considered as pathognomonic of MC since such cells may also be found in 10 to 30% of patients with parenchymal brain metastases. In solid tumors, therefore, the diagnosis of MC requires the association of CSF changes with clinical signs of MC.

The most frequent and specific CSF changes in MC are the increased protein and lowered glucose levels and the presence of neoplastic cells (Table 3.3). A nonspecific reaction of white blood cells is also frequent, consisting of a mixture of lymphocytes, polymorphonuclear cells, and, sometimes, macrophages. The CSF pressure is usually increased over 180 mm.

A significant elevation of polyamines, such as spermidine and spermine, has been observed by Rennert et al. (1977) in the CSF of children with ALL. The usefulness of these determinations in the early diagnosis of ML or for the monitoring of its treatment remains to be established.

Differential Diagnosis

In patients known to have a neoplasm, the main differential diagnoses of MC are brain metastases and infectious meningitis. In a number of patients, MC and brain metastases are associated. In pure leptomeningeal forms of MC, the onset is more insidious, and focal brain lesion signs are less frequent than in cerebral metastases. On the other hand, spinal root lesions are not seen, CSF glucose is normal, and neoplastic cells are found less frequently and in smaller amounts in brain metastases as compared with MC. Chronic or subacute meningoencephalitis caused by tuberculosis, yeast (mainly cryp-

TABLE 3.3. CSF changes in MC

References	Grain and Karr (1955)	Brucher and Cervós-Navarro (1960)	Vital et al. (1970)	Griffin et al. (1971)	Olson et al. (1974)	Little et al. (1974)
No. of cases examined	65 (literature review)	9	115 (literature review)	18	47	21
Protein	Increased: 44/48	Over 45 mg/100 ml: 6/9	Over 50 mg/100 ml: 73/115	Over 40 mg/100 ml: 16/18	Over 50 mg/100 ml: 43	Over 45 mg/100 ml: ,16/21
Glucose	Under 50 mg/100 ml: 15/25	Under 50 mg/100 ml: 4/5	—	Under 50 mg/100 ml: 8/18	Under 50 mg/100 ml: 36	Under 45 mg/100 ml: 16/21
Malignant cells	Found in 7; suspected in 18	Found in 3	Found in 33; suspected in 18	Found in 15/18	Found in 37	Found in 17/21
White blood cells	Increased in 28	Increased in 7/8	Over 10 cells/mm^3: 75/115	Increased in all CSF with malignant cells	Over 4 cells/mm^3: 36	Over 10 cells/mm^3: 10/21

tococcus neoformans), or sarcoidosis may be difficult to differentiate from MC. Tuberculous meningitis is the most common cause of low CSF glucose. Unlike in MC, CSF chloride concentration is decreased in tuberculous meningitis, and the patients are febrile.

Cryptococcal meningitis is rare in an unselected population but its frequency increases markedly in immunodepressed patients, especially those with lymphomas where MC is also frequent, reaching 29% in most recent reports (Bunn et al., 1976).

In patients with MC in whom mental syndromes are prominent, a diagnosis of encephalitis or metabolic encephalopathy is often made. A careful examination for the presence of neoplastic cells in the CSF should help to avoid such errors.

Treatment of Meningeal Carcinomatosis (MC)

The results achieved in MC in patients with leukemias and lymphomas or other solid tumors are considered separately.

Treatment of Meningeal Leukemia (ML)

The comparison of results achieved in the treatment of ML is somewhat difficult since studies may differ in patient selection, systemic chemotherapy regimens, and common definitions for cure and relapse. Since ML may be diagnosed in the absence of clinical signs by the presence of blasts in CSF, the length of remissions and the rate of relapse are obviously related to the frequency of lumbar punctures and techniques used for CSF examinations, which also differ from one study to another.

Treatment of Overt ML

Chemotherapy. Probably the best results in the treatment of overt ML were reported by Bleyer et al. (1976) with MTX given via an Ommaya reservoir. Two different regimens were used (either 12 mg/m^2 or 1 mg q. 12 hr × 6), both being repeated every 4 to 8 days for 8 weeks, and then monthly. The two regimens appeared equally effective, with a mean remission of more than 300 days and only one failure in 19 patients to achieve a remission. Neurotoxicity was considerably lower with the low-dosage schedule. The results previously achieved with intrathecal antifolics, reviewed by Sullivan et al. (1969), were less satisfactory. Although the remission rates were high (reaching 100% in some studies), medium or mean duration of remissions lasted less than 6 months. The difference between results reported in these studies and those achieved by Bleyer et al. (1976) is probably due to the omission of maintenance of intrathecal MTX in other trials.

Cytosine arabinoside (ara-C) was administered intrathecally by Wang and Pratt (1970) at dosages ranging from 5 to 70 mg/m² twice a week. Of 13 patients (11 with ALL and two with AML), seven responded to the treatment, but the mean duration of the remission was only 28 days. Band et al. (1973) have observed objective clinical improvements in six patients with ALL and three with AML after intrathecal administration of 4.5 to 73 mg ara-C/m² every 3 to 7 days. Only in three cases, however, was the count of blasts in the CSF lower than 2 cells/mm³ at the end of treatment.

A third drug, thio-tepa, has been used recently in the treatment of MC by Gutin et al. (1976) in doses from 1 to 10 mg/m² body surface area. Three patients with ALL had a complete response, four others had a partial response, and two failed to respond.

Substances that cross the blood-brain barrier have been administered systematically in the treatment of ML. Although they are not first-choice drugs, their use should be considered in cases where intrathecal treatments cannot be used or have failed.

Pyrimethamine, a potent folic acid antagonist, was administered by Geils et al. (1971) to two patients with AML and produced a 6- and 7-month remission of ML. BCNU has been used with some success by Nies et al. (1965) and Iriarte et al. (1966).

Corticosteroids, particularly dexamethasone, relieve signs of ML and may be recommended as emergency therapy when other treatments must be delayed for 1 or 2 days.

Radiotherapy. Radiotherapy used alone is of limited value in the treatment of overt ML. Cranial irradiation with 1,000 rads is ineffective; when extended to the whole craniospinal axis, it produced a remission of CSF abnormalities in 92%, but the mean duration was only 52 days (Sullivan et al., 1969). Sullivan et al. (1974) were able to prolong the mean duration of the remission to 216 days by increasing the dosage of craniospinal irradiations to 2,000 to 2,500 rads.

When radiotherapy is combined with intrathecal MTX, its benefit in the treatment of overt ML is uncertain. Thus the addition to the intrathecal MTX of a 1,000-rad irradiation of the spinal axis and a 2,500-rad irradiation of the cranium gives better results than the same chemotherapy alone when this chemotherapy is not maintained (Willoughby, 1974); but in a trial with continuing monthly intrathecal MTX administration, the addition of a 2,500-rad irradiation limited to the cranium was of no benefit (Duttera et al., 1973).

In summary: (1) Intrathecal MTX (possibly ara-C) produces a high rate (> 90%) of remissions in patients with overt ML, especially in ALL. (2) Maintenance of intrathecal MTX (possibly ara-C) is necessary. (3) Craniospinal irradiation alone cannot eradicate ML. (4) The benefit of the addition of craniospinal irradiation to intrathecal administration of MTX has been established only when intrathecal MTX is not maintained.

Prophylactic Treatment of ML

The so-called prophylactic treatment of ML has been prompted by poor long-term results achieved in the treatment of overt ML. The relative resistance of the leukemic blasts present in the CSF to both intrathecal chemotherapy and irradiation may be due to their low proliferation rate (Kuo et al., 1975). The slow rate of blastic proliferation in the subdural space may also account for the delay in separating the invasion of the subdural space by the leukemic cells from the development of overt ML. The following observations indicate that the penetration of neoplastic cells into the meninges may occur early in the development of the disease: (1) High white blood cell and low platelet counts at the time of diagnosis of acute leukemias have been correlated with subsequent apparition of ML (Table 3.4), suggesting that the passage of neoplastic blasts into CSF occurs early in the course of the disease. (2) Hyman et al. (1965) have observed that CNS leukemia and initial systemic disease have the same sensitivity or resistance to MTX. Intrathecal MTX may still be active in patients whose systemic disease, initially sensitive to MTX, becomes resistant to the drug. This indicates again that leukemic blasts infiltrate the leptomeninges in the early courses of acute leukemias.

First attempts to prevent ML were made by Melhorn et al. (1970), who gave only one intrathecal injection of amethopterin. This treatment was sufficient to delay significantly the development of CNS leukemia but not to reduce the rate of this complication.

A dramatic reduction of CNS relapse in ALL was reported in 1972 by Aur et al. after craniospinal irradiation with 2,400 rads (Table 3.5). One year later, this group (Aur et al., 1973) confirmed the efficacy of the irradiation treatment and showed that replacement of spinal radiotherapy by five intrathecal injections of MTX gave equally good results and reduced the

TABLE 3.4. *Factors in pathogenesis of CNS leukemia*

References	No. of cases (diagnosis)	Increase of white blood cells	Decrease of platelets	Organomegaly
West et al. (1972)	165 (ALL)	+ ($\leq 10^4$ vs. $> 10^4$)	+ ($\leq 5.10^4$ vs. $> 5.10^4$)	+ (Lymph nodes)
Pavlovsky et al. (1973)	228 (ALL and AML)	+ ($\leq 10^4$ vs. $> 5.10^4$)	N I	+ (Liver, spleen and lymph nodes)
Melhorn et al. (1970)	47 (46 ALL and 1 AML)	+ ($\leq 10^4$ vs. $> 10^4$)	N I	N I

+, Statistically significant correlation; N I, not investigated.

TABLE 3.5. Prophylactic treatment of ML

References	Treatments	Rate of MC
Aur et al. (1972)	Craniospinal irradiation with 2,400 rads;	2/45
	Untreated controls	32/49
Aur et al. (1973)	Craniospinal irradiation with 2,400 rads;	2/49
	Cranial irradiation with 2,400 rads + IT MTX	3/45
MRC Working Party (1973)	Cranial irradiation with 2,400 rads, spinal	
	Irradiation with 1,000 rads + IT MTX;	1/75
	controls	26/80
Jacquillat et al. (1973)	IT MTX	30/89
Sackmann-Muriel et al. (1974)	Cranial irradiation with 2,400 rads + IT MTX	1/56
		(After 17 mo.)
Mathé et al. (1975)	Cranial irradiation with 1,500 rads + IT MTX	
	and ara-C;	2/32
	Craniospinal irradiation with ± 1,500 rads	
	+ IT MTX;	3/26
	Cranial irradiation + IT MTX;	2/17
	IT MTX alone;	9/37
	IT MTX + IT ara-C;	0/2
	Irradiation alone;	3/3
	Untreated controls	26/76
Haghbin et al. (1975)	IT MTX via Ommaya reservoir	
	(also given throughout maintenance)	4/70

myelotoxicity. Excellent results were also reported by the MRC Working Party on Leukemia of Childhood (1973) by using cranial irradiation (2,400 rads) combined with spinal radiotherapy (1,000 rads) and monthly intrathecal MTX. In 1974, Sackmann-Muriel et al. fully confirmed the results of Aur et al. (1973). Mathé et al. (1975) successively used several prophylactic treatments detailed in Table 3.5 and reported favorable results for several combinations. Table 3.6 shows pooled results of patients who received reasonably comparable treatments. These combined results indicate that two treatments, craniospinal irradiation with 2,400 rads and cranial irradiation with 2,400 rads plus five intrathecal injections of MTX, are able to reduce the rate of ML to 5%. MTX used alone seems to be less active (Nesbit et al., 1977) except in the studies of Haghbin et al. (1975) and Haghbin and Galicich (1977) where MTX was given through the Ommaya reservoir and where systemic chemotherapy included BCNU. Intraventricular chemotherapy may indeed be more effective against CNS leukemia than treatment given by lumbar puncture (Bleyer and Poplack, 1977).

In ALL, the dramatic drop of ML is one of the major steps toward the cure which may be expected in almost 50% of treated children. In AML, however, where chemotherapy is less effective and the survival considerably shorter, the prophylaxis of ML is not systematically used, although 2,400-rad craniospinal irradiation can produce CNS relapse (Dahl et al., 1976). The

TABLE 3.6. *Reduction of the rate of relapse of CNS leukemia by three different prophylactic treatments*

Reference	Craniospinal irradiation (2,400 rads)	Cranial irradiation (2,400 rads) + IT MTX	IT MTX alone
Aur et al. (1972)	2/45	—	—
Aur et al. (1973)	2/49	3/45	—
Jacquillat et al. (1973)	—	—	30/89
Sackmann-Muriel et al. (1974)	—	1/56	—
Mathé et al. (1975)	—	2/17	9/37
Haghbin et al. (1975)	—	—	4/70
Total	4/94 (4.3%)	6/118 (5.1%)	Variable

use of CNS prophylaxis has been recently advocated by Renoux et al. (1977) in adults with AML, but the limited number of patients treated in this study does not allow for any definitive conclusion.

Solid Tumor MC

The involvement of leptomeninges in patients with solid primary tumors indicates poor response to antineoplastic treatments. However, encouraging results have been obtained in primary tumors most sensitive to radio- and chemotherapy. In the study by Griffin et al. (1971), 13 patients with lymphomatous leptomeningitis received intrathecal MTX by a variety of schedules; eight were also treated by whole-brain irradiation (doses varying from 300 rads in 3 days to 3,000 rads in 12 days). In seven patients in whom therapy was usually combined, the cytology and chemistry of CSF and the clinical status improved enough to allow the patients to be discharged. However, all the patients in this study died within 20 months.

In the study by Olson et al. (1974), five of 14 patients with lymphomatous MC who received intrathecal chemotherapy (MTX or ara-C) and/or radiation improved. Two other patients improved, one after systemic chemotherapy and another after irradiation of the base of the brain. Complete responses have been reported in three of six patients with lymphoma and CNS involvement after high doses of systemically administered MTX (1 to 7.5 mg/m^2) plus citrovorum factor (Zuckerman et al., 1976). Seven of 14 patients reported by Bunn et al. (1976) with lymphomatous leptomeningitis had a complete disappearance of malignant cells from CSF after irradiation and intrathecal chemotherapy.

In the study by Olson et al. (1974), six of 18 patients with breast carcinoma responded to radiotherapy or intrathecal chemotherapy, or both; three responders survived 9 months, 1 year, and 1½ years, respectively. Three of five women with breast cancer and MC who were treated in this hospital by radio- and chemotherapy responded to treatment, the longest survival being 3 years (Hildebrand and Debusscher, 1977). Other data (Yap et al., 1977) also indicate that fairly aggressive therapy, continuing intrathecal chemotherapy, and irradiation prolong the duration and improve the quality of survival in patients with MC secondary to breast carcinoma.

In MC complicating other solid tumors, responses to treatment have been reported only occasionally (Heatfield and Williams, 1956; Bender, 1974), but the results are generally disappointing and death usually occurs within a few weeks or months.

METASTATIC LESIONS OF PERIPHERAL NERVES

Neoplastic cells may injure any part of the peripheral nervous system (PNS), producing pain, depression of deep reflexes, muscle atrophy, and motor and sensory deficits. The most frequently injured structures are cranial nerves and nerve plexus.

Cranial Nerves

Lesions of cranial nerves are common in patients with skull metastases, the nerves being injured as they leave the cranium. Involvement of cranial nerves is primarily seen in cancers with bone metastases, such as breast, prostate, thyroid, kidney, and lung carcinoma. Palsies of facial and oculomotor nerves are most commonly seen. Radiotherapy is effective and may restore nervous functions when promptly initiated.

Differential diagnosis must be made with parenchymal brainstem metastases and carcinomatous or infectious (cryptococcus neoformans) meningitis. In patients with cancer, these causes of cranial nerve palsies are less frequent than lesions caused by skull metastases (see Table 1 in the preface to this volume). In addition, in all of these diseases neurological signs are seldom limited to cranial nerve abnormalities. Radiation and chemotherapy may also produce cranial nerve lesions (see Chapters 4 and 5).

Finally, causes not related to cancer, such as Bell palsy of the facial nerve, diabetes, and vitamin deficiencies, must also be considered in the differential diagnosis.

Plexus Lesions

Metastatic involvement of the brachial plexus occurs mainly in patients with breast and lung carcinomas. Such lesions have been observed by Son (1967) in 15 of 347 cases of lung cancer and seven of 278 patients with breast carcinoma. Among the patients with lung cancer, 14 also had palsies of recurrent laryngeal nerve and five of phrenic nerve. The onset of metastatic involvement of brachial plexus is progressive. First symptoms consist of pain, often severe, radiating through the upper limb. Pain is followed by depression of deep reflexes, weakness, predominantly in distal segments, amyotrophy, and objective sensory disorders.

Irradiation may be effective. Nisce and Chu (1968) have treated 47 patients with brachial plexus lesions due to breast cancer metastases with 3,000 to 3,500 rads. Pain relief was complete in 25.5% and partial in 49%. Motor and/or sensory recovery was excellent in 15% of cases, where restoration of neurological functions was observed, and partial in 32%. Similarly, favorable results were reported by Son (1967), especially for irradiation doses of more than 3,000 rads.

The differential diagnosis of metastatic lesions of brachial plexus may be difficult in women with breast cancer previously treated by irradiations on the brachial plexus area (see Chapter 5).

The features of the postirradiation lesions of brachial plexus may indeed be very similar to those due to neoplastic infiltration. The nerves of the lower limbs are most commonly injured by the neoplasm invading the pelvis, mainly the squamous epithelioma of the cervix uteri.

REFERENCES

Aaronson, A. G., Hajdu, S. L., and Melamed, H. R. (1975): Spinal fluid cytology during chemotherapy of leukemia of the central nervous system in children. *Am. J. Clin. Pathol.*, 63:528–537.

Altrocchi, P. H., and Eckman, P. B. (1973): Meningeal carcinomatosis and blindness. *J. Neurol. Neurosurg. Psychiatry*, 36:206–210.

Amiel, J. L., and Droz, J. P. (1976): Lymphocytose rachidienne au cours de la leucémie lymphocytaire chronique. *Nouv. Presse Med.*, 5:94.

Ardichvili, D., Henneaux, J., and Musin, L. (1971): Carcinomatose méningée à localisation exclusivement spinale et à point de départ inconnu. *Arch. Med. Brux.*, 27: 655–663.

Aur, R. J. A., Simone, J. V., Hustu, H. O., and Verzosa, M. S. (1972): A comparative study of central nervous system irradiation and intensive chemotherapy early in remission of childhood lymphocytic leukemia. *Cancer*, 29:381–391.

Aur, R. J. A., Hustu, H. O., Verzosa, M. S., Wood, A., and Simone, J. V. (1973): Comparison of two methods of preventing central nervous system leukemia. *Blood*, 42:349–357.

Band, P. R., Holland, J. F., Bernard, J., Weil, M., Walker, M., and Rall, D. (1973): Treatment of central nervous system leukemia with intrathecal cytosine arabinoside. *Cancer*, 32:744–748.

Bender, R. A. (1974): Meningeal carcinomatosis: Treatment with intrathecal methotrexate. *Oncology*, 30:328–333.

Bleyer, W. A., Poplack, D. G., Ziegler, J. L., Leventhal, B. G., Ommaya, A. K., and Chabner, B. A. (1976): "Concentration time" methotrexate therapy of meningeal leukemia via a subcutaneous reservoir: A controlled clinical trial. *ASCO Abstr.*, p. 253.

Bleyer, W. A., and Poplack, J. G. (1977): Intraventricular vs intralumbar methotrexate for central nervous system leukemia: Prolonged remission with the Ommaya reservoir. *AACR Abstr.*, p. 103.

Brucher, J. M., and Cervós-Navarro, J. (1960): La carcinomatose méningée—Etude anatomoclinique de 11 cas. *Acta Neurol. Psychiatr. Belg.*, 60:368–395.

Bunn, P. A., Schein, P. S., Banks, P. M., and DeVita, V. T. (1976): CNS complications in patients with diffuse histiocytic and undifferentiated lymphoma: Leukemia revisited. *Blood,* 47:3–10.

Dahl, G., Simone, J., Hustu, H. O., and Mason, E. W. (1976): Preventive CNS irradiation in acute myelogenous leukemia. *Blood,* 48:961.

Danis, P., and Brihaye-van Geertruyden, M. (1952): Névrite optique rétrobulbaire bilatérale par métastases cancéreuses dans les gaines arachnoïdiennes. *Acta Neurol. Psychiatr. Belg.,* 52:345–359.

Dawson, D. M., Rosenthal, D. S., and Moloney, W. C. (1973): Neurological complications of acute leukemia in adults: Changing rate. *Acta Int. Med.,* 79:541–544.

Duttera, M. J., Bleyer, W. A., Pomeroy, T. C., Leventhal, C. M., and Leventhal, B. (1973): Irradiation, methotrexate toxicity, and the treatment of meningeal leukemia. *Lancet,* ii:703–707.

Evans, A. E., Gilbert, E. S., and Zandstra, R. (1970): The increasing incidence of central nervous system leukemia in children. *Cancer,* 26:404–409.

Evans, D. I. K., O'Rourke, C., and Morris Jones, P. (1974): The cerebrospinal fluid in acute leukemia of childhood: Studies with cytocentrifuge. *J. Clin. Pathol.,* 27:226–230.

Fischer-Williams, M., Bosanquet, F. D., and Daniel, P. M. (1955): Carcinomatosis of the meninges. A report of three cases. *Brain,* 78:42–58.

Geils, G. F., Scott, C. W., Jr., Bangh, C. M., and Butterworth, C. E., Jr. (1971): Treatment of meningeal leukemia with pyrimethamine. *Blood,* 38:131–137.

Grain, G. O., and Karr, J. P. (1955): Diffuse leptomeningeal carcinomatosis. Clinical and pathologic characteristics. *Neurology,* 5:706–722.

Griffin, J., Thompson, R. W., Mitchinson, M. J., Kiewiet, J. C., and Welland, F. H. (1971): Lymphomatous leptomeningitis. *Am. J. Med.,* 51:200–208.

Gutin, P. H., Weiss, H. D., Wiernik, P. H., and Walker, M. D. (1976): Intrathecal N, N′, N″,-triethylenethiophosphoramine [Thio-Tepa (NSC-6396)] in the treatment of malignant meningeal disease. Phase I-II study. *Cancer,* 38:1471–1475.

Haghbin, M., Tan, C. T. C., Clarkson, B. D., Mike, V., Burchenal, J. H., and Murphy, M. L. (1975): Treatment of acute lymphoblastic leukemia in children with prophylactic intrathecal methotrexate and intensive systemic chemotherapy. *Cancer Res.,* 35:807–811.

Haghbin, M., and Galicich, J. (1977): A long-term follow-up of Ommaya reservoir for prophylaxis and treatment of central nervous system leukemia. *ASCO Abstr.,* p. 342.

Heatfield, K. W. G., and Williams, J. R. B. (1956): Carcinomatosis of the meninges. Some clinical and pathological aspects. *Br. Med. J.,* 6:328–330.

Hildebrand, J., and Debusscher, L. (1977): Meningeal carcinomatosis. In: *Recent Advances in Cancer Treatment,* edited by H. J. Tagnon and M. J. Staquet, pp. 241–253. Raven Press, New York.

Hyman, C. B., Bogle, J. M., Brubaker, G. C. A., Williams, K., and Hammond, D. (1965): Central nervous system involvement by leukemia and description of clinical and laboratory manifestations. *Blood,* 25:1–2.

Kuo, A. H., Yataganas, X., Galilich, J. H., Fried, J., and Clarkson, B. D. (1975): Proliferative kinetics of central nervous system leukemia. *Cancer,* 36:232–239.

Little, J. R., Dale, A. J. D., and Okazaki, H. (1974): Meningeal carcinomatosis. *Arch. Neurol.,* 30:138–143.

Mathé, G., Pouillart, P., and Schwarzenberg, L. (1975): Meningeal localization of acute leukemias. *Acta Neuropathol. (Berl.) [Suppl.],* VI:235–239.

Melhorn, D. K., Gross, S., Fisher, B. J., and Newman, A. J. (1970): Studies on the use of "prophylactic" intrathecal amethopterin in childhood leukemia. *Blood,* 36:55–60.

MRC Working Party on Leukaemia in Childhood (1973): Treatment of acute lymphoblastic leukaemia: Effect of "prophylactic" therapy against central nervous system leukaemia. *Br. Med. J.,* 2:381–384.

Nesbit, M., Donaldson, M., Ortega, J., Hittle, R., Hammond, D., Weiner, J., and Sather, H. (1977): Influence of an isolated central nervous system relapse on subsequent marrow relapse in childhood lymphoblastic leukemia. *AARC Abstr.,* p. 143.

Nies, B. A., Thomas, L. B., and Freireich, E. J. (1965): Meningeal leukemia: A follow-up study. *Cancer,* 18:546–553.

Nisce, L. Z., and Chu, F. C. H. (1968): Radiation therapy of brachial plexus syndrome from breast cancer. *Radiology*, 91:1022–1025.

Olson, M. E., Chernik, N. L., and Posner, J. B. (1974): Infiltration of the leptomeninges in systemic cancer. *Arch. Neurol.*, 30:122–137.

Parsons, M. (1972): The spinal form of carcinomatous meningitis. *Q. J. Med.* [*New Series*], XLI:509–519.

Pavlovsky, S., Eppinger-Helft, M., and Sackmann-Muriel, F. (1973): Factors that influence the appearance of central nervous system leukemia. *Blood*, 42:935–938.

Peterson, B. A., and Bloomfield, C. D. (1977): Asymptomatic central nervous system leukemia in adults with acute non-lymphocytic leukemia in extended remission. *ASCO Abstr.*, p. 341.

Pochedly, C. (1975): Neurologic manifestation in acute leukemia. *N.Y. State J. Med.*, 75:I. 575–580; II. 715–721; III. 878–882.

Rennert, O. M., Lawson, D. L., Shukla, J. B., and Miale, T. D. (1977): Cerebrospinal fluid polyamine monitoring in central nervous system leukemia. *Clin. Chim. Acta*, 75:365–369.

Renoux, M., Dhermy, D., Bernard, J. F., Brousse, N., Henin, D., Amar, M., and Boivin, P. (1977): Localisations cérébro-méningées des leucémies aiguës myéloblastiques de l'adulte. Etude clinique et anatomo-pathologique de 15 cas. *Nouv. Rev. Fr. Hematol.*, 18:23–34.

Sackmann-Muriel, F., Pavlovky, S., Penalvez, J. A., Hidalgo, G., Cebrian-Bonesana, A., Eppinger-Helft, M., de Macchi, G. H., and Pavlovsky, A. (1974): Evaluation of induction of remission, intensification and central nervous system prophylactic treatment in acute lymphoblastic leukemia. *Cancer*, 34:418–426.

Schwartz, J. H., Canellos, G. P., Young, R. C., and DeVita, V. T. (1975): Meningeal leukemia in the blastic phase of chronic granulocytic leukemia. *Am. J. Med.*, 59:819–828.

Son, Y. H. (1967): Effectiveness of irradiation therapy in peripheral neuropathy caused by malignant disease. *Cancer*, 20:1447.

Sullivan, M. P., Vietti, T. J., Fernbach, D. J., Griffith, K. M., Haddy, T. B., and Watkins, W. L. (1969): Clinical investigations in treatment of meningeal leukemia: Radiation therapy regimens vs. conventional intrathecal methotrexate. *Blood*, 34:301–319.

Sullivan, M. P., Humphrey, G. B., Vietti, T. J., Haggard, M. E., and Lee, E. (1974): Superiority of conventional intrathecal methotrexate therapy with maintenance over intensive intrathecal methotrexate therapy, unmaintained, or radiotherapy (2000–2500 rads tumor dose) in treatment of meningeal leukemia. *Cancer*, 35:1066–1073.

Vital, C., Bruno-Martin, F., Henry, P., Bergouignan, M., and Leger, H. (1970): La carcinomatose méningée. *Bord. Med.*, 3:2927–2944.

Wang, J. J., and Pratt, C. B. (1970): Intrathecal arabinosyl-cytosine in meningeal leukemia. *Cancer*, 25:531–534.

West, R. J., Graham-Pole, J., Hardisty, R. M., and Pike, M. C. (1972): Factors in pathogenesis of central nervous system leukemia. *Br. Med. J.*, 3:311–314.

Willoughby, M. L. N. (1974): Treatment of overt meningeal leukaemia. *Lancet*, i:363.

Yap, B. S., Yap, H. Y., Benjamin, R. S., Blumenchein, G. R., Hart, J. S., and Bodey, G. P. (1977): Treatment of meningeal carcinomatosis. *ASCO Abstr.*, p. 287.

Zuckerman, K. S., Skarin, A. T., Pitman, S. W., Rosenthal, D. S., and Canellos, G. P. (1976): High dose methotrexate with citrovorum factor in the treatment of advanced non-Hodgkin's lymphoma. *Blood*, 48:983.

Chapter 4

Neurotoxic Effects of Drugs Used in Cancer Chemotherapy

In addition to drugs used frequently but not exclusively in cancer patients (such as steroids, which produce psychosis and myopathy), numerous specifically antineoplastic substances have neurological side effects. They may injure the nervous system at all levels, producing a variety of syndromes (Table 4.1). We consider (a) encephalopathies, (b) cerebellar dysfunctions, (c) injuries of the meninges, spinal cord, and/or nerve roots, and (d) lesions of cranial and peripheral nerves.

TABLE 4.1. *Neurological syndromes caused by anticancer drugs*

Encephalopathies

    Antifolates: MTX, DDMP
    Antipyrimidines: Ara-C, 5-FU, 5-azacytidine
    Procarbazine
    Alkylating agents: NH_2, chlorambucil, cyclophosphamide,
                     phenylalamine mustard, DTIC (?)
    Vinca alkaloids: VCR
    L-Asparaginase
    OpDDD

Cerebellar Dysfunctions

    5-FU
    Procarbazine
    BCNU
    OpDDD
    Treatment of CNS leukemia (MTX ?)

Injuries of Meninges, Spinal Cord, and/or Nerve Roots

    Thio-tepa (?)
    MTX
    Ara-C

Lesions of Peripheral and Cranial Nerves

    Vinca alkaloids: VCR, vindesine, vinblastine, formyl leurosine
    Procarbazine
    VP 16–213
    5-Azacytidine
    Cis-platinum
    OpDDD
    BCNU (optic neuritis); CCNU (retinal abnormalities ?)

ENCEPHALOPATHIES

Brain dysfunctions, including psychiatric disorders and seizures, have been observed in patients treated with a large variety of drugs (Table 4.1).

Antifolates

Methotrexate

Methotrexate (MTX), which inhibits dihydrofolate reductase, is an analog of folic acid. Its activity may be reversed by the administration of the latter. To reach the neoplastic cells located in the meninges or in the brain, MTX is usually given intrathecally. Under certain circumstances, however, such as concomitant irradiation of the brain or administration of high systemic doses, MTX may cross the blood-brain barrier. In addition, high doses of intravenous MTX given simultaneously with intrathecal or intraventricular injections enhance the concentrations of the drug in cerebrospinal fluid (CSF) (Creaven et al., 1977).

Encephalopathies caused by MTX have been described in two clinical situations: (1) in patients with brain tumors receiving intraventricular injections of MTX, and (2) after prophylactic or curative treatments of meningeal leukemia.

(1) Necrotizing encephalopathies following intraventricular administration of MTX are rare. Three such cases were reported by Shapiro et al. (1973), all clinically characterized by acute bilateral cerebral and upper brainstem dysfunction rapidly progressing to mutism and decerebrate posturing. In this study, total doses of MTX administered via ventricular catheter ranged from 86 to 190 mg. The onset of encephalopathies was observed 3 to 5 months after the initiation of intrathecal MTX and 10, 13, and 42 months after brain irradiation with 3,600 to 6,000 rads. Four other cases have been reported by Norrell et al. (1974). Their patients developed signs of encephalopathy 3 to 15 months after the administration of MTX, when the dosage of the drug given intrathecally reached 130 to 600 mg. All patients received brain irradiation (1,500 to 4,560 rads) 26 to 67 months prior to the first signs of encephalopathy.

At autopsy, all patients had a severe leukoencephalopathy involving mainly the central white matter of cerebral hemispheres. These lesions of coagulation necrosis were particularly striking in periventricular areas. In all patients reported by Norrell et al. and in one case of the Shapiro et al. study, blood vessel lesions were absent. Because nervous system lesions had a periventricular distribution and because vessels were not injured in all cases, the pathogenesis of this leukoencephalopathy was attributed to MTX rather than to radiotherapy. Shapiro and co-workers considered that ventricular obstruction is necessary to enhance the local neurotoxicity of MTX. Norrell and his associates also believed that this mechanism had favored the development of the leukoencephalopathies, although no tumor had been found at autopsy in one of their patients.

(2) Encephalopathies of patients treated for central nervous system (CNS) leukemia have been reported under different designations (Table 4.2). These diseases were observed after prolonged treatments with systemic and intrathecal MTX, but a number of these patients also received brain radiotherapy and other potentially neurotoxic drugs (Table 4.2). Although the treatment of CNS leukemia is considered the main factor in the pathogenesis of these encephalopathies, the precise mechanism of their etiology is not fully understood. Therefore, one cannot be sure that all the cases reported in the studies summarized in Table 4.2 represent the same disease.

The role of high doses of systemic MTX in the pathogenesis of these encephalopathies clearly appears in the study of Aur et al. (1975), in which severe encephalopathy developed in nine of 20 children who received 50 to 80 mg MTX/m^2 i.v. weekly. This complication, however, was not observed in the three other arms of the trial, including in children who received 20 to 30 mg of MTX/m^2 i.v. weekly. However, not all leukemic patients suffering from encephalopathy received high doses or prolonged treatment with MTX.

Clinical features of these encephalopathies are similar in different reports. The most frequent signs observed are drooling, confusion, irritability, and somnolence, which may lead to coma and death. Ataxia and spasticity are frequently mentioned. Seizures or focal neurological deficits are present in approximately 25% of cases. The EEG invariably shows diffuse, often asymmetrical slow waves. Brain isotope scan and intracarotid angiographies are usually normal.

Pathological features reported in various studies show some discrepancies. In the only case of Kay et al. (1972) in which the pathological examination was performed, the authors stressed the importance of infarcted areas. In other studies, vessel lesions, although frequent, were not always present. The most characteristic lesion consisted of multiple disseminated focal necroses with an astrocytic reaction. These lesions were found in the white matter, but unlike those in necrotizing encephalopathies following intrathecal administration of MTX, they were not limited to the periventricular areas.

Inflammatory reactions, infectious agents, or infiltrations by leukemic blasts were absent in all cases examined. In some cases, intracerebral calcifications have been observed (Borns and Rancier, 1974; Flament-Durand et al., 1975; Meadows and Evans, 1976).

Treatment consists of discontinuation of potentially neurotoxic chemotherapy, especially of MTX. Kay et al. (1972) have attributed partial regressions of clinical features to the administration of folic and folinic acids.

TABLE 4.2. Leukoencephalopathies in patients treated for CNS-leukemia

Reference	Encephalopathy	No. of cases	Main symptoms and signs	Pathology: main features	Possibly neurotoxic treatment MTX (i.t.)	Other
Kay et al. (1972)	Encephalopathy in AL associated with MTX	7	Confusion, tremor, ataxia, irritability, drooling, somnolence, coma	Infarcted areas (1 case examined)	Prolonged i.t. and p.o. MTX given to all pat.	Cranial RT given to 3 pat. before and to 2 pat. after onset of encephalopathy; i.t. ara-C given to 2 pat.
McIntosh and Aspnes (1973)	Encephalopathy following CNS prophylaxis	6 (of 33)	Lethargy, somnolence, irritability, seizures, tremor, ataxia		5 injections of i.t. MTX	Cranial RT (2,000–2,500 rads) and VCR; i.v. MTX 2×/wk given to all pat.
Hendin et al. (1974)	Parenchymatous degeneration of CNS in leukemia	(a) 1 (b) 22	(a) Dementia, seizures, ataxia, spasticity (b) Without clinical signs or symptoms	Fibrillary gliosis	(a) i.t. MTX (b) 14 pat. received i.t. MTX	(a) VCR i.v., 2,100 rads CNS-RT, i.t. ara-C (b) 7 pat.: 600–3,000 rads; 3 pat.: i.t. ara-C
Rubinstein et al. (1975)	Disseminated necrotizing leukoencephalopathy	5	Lethargy, dysphagia, irritability, focal deficit	Multifocal coagulative necroses in white matter	All pat. received i.t. MTX, some systemic MTX	All pat. received cranial RT, i.v. VCR, and i.t. ara-C
Price and Jamieson (1975)	Subacute leukoencephalopathy in childhood leukemia	13 (of 231)	Mental changes, seizures, ataxia, spasticity, focal deficits	Multiple necrotic pain, astrocytosis in white matter	All pat. received i.t. MTX	All pat. received RT and i.v. MTX during RT
Meadows and Evans (1976)		4 (of 23)	Dementia, seizures, spastic quadriplegia or paraplegia	White matter gliosis	All had i.v. MTX plus oral MTX in 2 cases	Three received RT; all pat. received VCR, and 2 ara-C

Abbreviations: AL, acute leukemia; pat., patient; ara-C, cytosine arabinoside; MTX, methotrexate; VCR, vincristine; RT, radiotherapy; i.t., intrathecal; p.o., per os; i.v., intravenous.

Methodichlorophen

Methodichlorophen (DDMP) acts as an antifolate, but its ability to inhibit dihydrofolate reductase is weak compared to MTX. In addition, DDMP inhibits the growth of MTX-resistant cells; it is lipophylic and reaches high concentrations in the brain and CSF. Severe headaches, haziness, and confusion have been reported, particularly in patients receiving 3 mg/kg body weight or more (Price et al., 1975).

Antipyrimidines

Cytosine-arabinoside (ara-C), which does not cross the blood-brain barrier, has been administered intrathecally to leukemia patients usually also treated with MTX. In some of them, leukoencephalopathies subsequently developed. However, the role of ara-C in their pathogenesis remains uncertain because of concomitant treatment with other chemotherapeutic agents.

5-Fluorouracil (5-FU) crosses the blood-brain barrier easily; it has a well-known toxicity for the cerebellum, but mild encephalopathies have been observed occasionally. Of 18 patients with cerebellar ataxia reported by Moertel et al. (1964), two complained of mild loss of memory and slowness of thought. Two other cases of confusion and mental changes were observed by Greenwald (1976) after weekly intravenous administration of 5-FU. Both patients became fully alert when chemotherapy was stopped.

5-Azacytidine has been used by Levi and Wiernik (1976) in leukemia patients. Eight of 17 patients experienced, in addition to the signs of peripheral neuropathy, deterioration of mental status, irritability, confusion, and lethargy.

Procarbazine

Procarbazine is a derivative of monoamine oxidase inhibitors; the mechanism of its antineoplastic activity is complex.

Cerebral toxicity may manifest itself as lassitude, sedation, or drowsiness. In rare instances, stupor has been observed (Brunner and Young, 1965; Stolinsky et al., 1970; DeConti, 1971).

When procarbazine is given per os, CNS symptoms appear for daily doses of more than 150 to 200 mg. Procarbazine crosses the blood-brain barrier easily, and chronic administration may inhibit brain monoamine oxidase. One should be warned, therefore, against the association of procarbazine with the inhibitors of monoamine oxidase.

Procarbazine also has a synergistic sedative effect when given together with barbiturates and phenothiazines. In clinical use, the neurotoxicity of procarbazine is seldom a limiting factor when the drug is given per os. In intravenous treatments using high doses of procarbazine (up to 1,000 mg/m^2 body surface), however, somnolence and lethargy are frequent and restrict the amounts which may be administered by this route (Chabner et al., 1973).

Alkylating Agents

Alkylating agents, which possess one or more chloroethyl groups, act primarily on DNA by forming bridges between the two DNA strands.

Nitrogen Mustard

Nitrogen mustard (NH_2) is the prototype of the alkylating agents; its neurotoxicity is rare when the drug is given systemically. However, when high doses (such as 0.9 mg/kg $\times$ 3) were given to patients with temporary aortic occlusion, drowsiness, confusion, and disorientation progressing to coma and death occurred in four of 18 patients (Cliford et al., 1963). More recently, a severe cerebral toxicity was reported by Bethlenfalvay and Bergin (1972) in a patient with Hodgkin disease treated with usual (0.4 mg/kg) doses of NH_2. Two almost identical and reversible episodes, characterized by fever, grand mal seizures, and coma, developed in this 35-year-old man within the week following the second and third doses of NH_2. Brain tissue appeared under increased pressure. CSF contained 517 cells (54% of polymorphonuclear and 46% of lymphocytes), and protein was 101 mg/100 ml. The patient died 8 years later; focal areas of gliosis with loss of neurons were found at autopsy.

Alkylating agents are more frequently neurotoxic when administered by intracarotid regional perfusion. The interest of these neurological side effects is rather historic since the intracarotid route of drug administration is no longer used in the treatment of brain tumors. Jacksonian convulsions, confusion, contralateral hemiplegia, coma, and death due to progressive cerebral degeneration have been frequently observed with NH_2 and another alkylating agent, phenylalanine mustard (French et al., 1952; Ariel, 1961). This neurotoxicity may be decreased when the total doses of NH_2 are limited to 14 to 16 mg (Owens and Hatiboglu, 1961).

Chlorambucil

Milder forms of brain toxicity were reported after systemic administration of this alkylating agent. Convulsive disorders and a comatose state, which disappeared within a few days, were observed in a 2½-year-old child after accidental ingestion of about 70 mg chlorambucil (Wolfson and Olney, 1957). Transitory lethargy, ataxia, and hyperactivity occurred in another 2-year-old after ingestion of 1.5 mg chlorambucil/kg body weight (Green and Naiman, 1968).

Cyclophosphamide

Sensations of dizziness were produced regularly in five patients at each intraventricular push of 500 mg cyclophosphamide (Tashima, 1975).

Dimethyltriazono Imidazole Carboxamide (DTIC)

Occasional neurological disorders, such as epileptic seizures (Gams and Carpenter, 1974), cerebral hemorrhage without thrombocytopenia (Gerner et al., 1973), and severe dementia (Paterson and McPherson, 1977), have been observed in patients treated with dimethyltriazono imidazole carboxamide (DTIC).

The relationship between the drug and the neurological lesions remains speculative. DTIC has the structural characteristics of purine antagonists but the biological activity of alkylating agents. It crosses the blood-brain barrier to some extent.

Vincristine

Neurotoxicity is the main side effect of vincristine (VCR). VCR does not readily cross the blood-brain barrier, and its toxicity is usually limited to the peripheral nerves. Intrathecal injection of VCR causes death with marked neural changes characterized by clumped Nissl substance and acidophylic crystals (Schochet et al., 1968). CNS toxicity is rare when VCR is given intravenously; but seizures (Kleinknecht et al., 1967), mental changes, confusion and speech difficulties (Costa et al., 1962), delirium, slow mentation and hallucinations (Reitmeier et al., 1964), and coma (Slater et al., 1969, Lôo and Zittoun, 1969; Whittaker et al., 1973; Jean et al., 1976) have been described.

In some patients treated with VCR, comas were attributed to hyponatremia resulting from inappropriate secretion of antidiuretic hormone. Abnormal secretion of antidiuretic hormone may be due either to a direct action on the CNS (hypothalamus, neurohypophyseal tract, or posterior pituitary) or to derangements in neuronal input from peripheral volume receptors (Slater et al., 1969; Whittaker et al., 1973). In other cases, however, the mechanism of coma after VCR therapy remains obscure. Death does not usually occur, and autopsies of patients who died subsequently were unhelpful. More recently, Rosemberg (1974) described cerebral ischemic infarctions due to arteriolar thrombosis and necrosis in the brain of a child who died 26 days after the onset of an acute encephalopathy attributed to VCR therapy. Identical lesions were also observed by Jean et al. (1976) in two children who died from acute encephalopathy attributed to VCR, although both patients also received intrathecal MTX. Seizures attributed to VCR therapy have been observed mainly in children. Their incidence in 230 patients studied by

Kleinknecht et al. (1967) was 4.5%. The convulsions are of grand mal type, usually occur 2 to 6 days after VCR administration, and responded in part to treatment, particularly to diazepam. Of 11 patients with seizures described in Kleinknecht's study, seven had other neurological abnormalities, such as hemiplegia (seen in four cases), astereognosis, paraplegia, and paralysis of the abducens nerve.

L-Asparaginase

L-Asparaginase is an enzyme that catalyzes the hydrolysis of *l'*asparagine and can deprive this essential amino acid from cells, such as leukemic blasts, which do not possess the ability to synthetize *l'*asparagine.

Clinical use of L-asparaginase is limited by a series of side effects, e.g., allergic reactions, coagulopathy, pancreatitis, hepatotoxicity, and CNS toxicity. Neurotoxicity is frequent (Table 4.3), consisting of a more or less severe change in personality and consciousness, ranging from mild confusion, disorientation, somnolence, or lethargy to acute delirium, stupor, and even coma (Haskell et al., 1969*a,b;* Oettgen et al., 1970; Moure et al., 1970; Ohnuma et al., 1970; Land et al., 1972). Rare cases of parkinsonism have been reported (Storti and Quaglino, 1970). The frequency of CNS toxicity after asparaginase therapy is summarized in Table 4.3 (Weiss et al., 1974), usually varying from 25 to 50%. Asparaginase neurotoxicity was not observed in some studies (Jacquillat et al., 1970), and the authors have attributed this absence of side effects to methods used for drug purification; however, this opinion has not been confirmed. In most but not all cases (Table 4.3), the encephalopathy caused by asparaginase treatment is accompanied by EEG changes consisting of a reduced frequency of basal rhythm and

TABLE 4.3. *Signs of L-asparaginase neurotoxicity[a]*

		Disorder in quality or level of consciousness			Abnormal EEG during therapy
References	Dose	Total	Mild	Severe	
Haskell et al. (1969[b])	200 IU/kg/day	18/35[b]	13/35	5/35	
Oettgen et al. (1970)	1,000–5,000 IU/kg/day	71/156[c] 48/147[d]			
Moure et al. (1970)	600–400,000 IU/m²/day	14/23			20/23
Ohnuma et al. (1970)	200–40,000 IU/kg (single, daily, or weekly)	18/45	11/45	7/45	
Land et al. (1972)	200 IU/kg (variable schedule)	26/123	15/123	11/123	19/26

[a] From Weiss et al., 1974.
[b] Figures are no. of cases/no. of patients.
[c] Adults.
[d] Children.

presence of diffuse slow waves. Signs of brain dysfunction may appear during the first days of treatment. These are to some extent related to the daily dosage of the drug, tend to occur more often in adults than in children, and are reversible. In patients with severe encephalopathies, the administration of asparaginase must be discontinued; in milder cases, however, changes in the dosage or schedule allow the continuation of treatment.

The mechanisms of brain dysfunction in asparaginase treatment remain unclear. Since asparaginase does not easily cross the blood-brain barrier, it is unlikely that it acts directly on brain metabolism. Increase of blood ammonia due to hepatotoxicity is responsible for mental changes observed after asparaginase treatment. However, the correlation between the degree of brain dysfunction and blood ammonia levels is not absolute. Other mechanisms have also been considered (Haskell et al., 1969*b*), such as alteration of brain metabolism by increased levels of *l*-aspartic and *l*-glutamic acids or interference with brain protein synthesis due to depletion of *l*-asparagine. The last mechanism has been postulated to cause the organic brain syndrome which occasionally occurs 1 week after discontinuation of asparaginase treatment (Ohnuma et al., 1970).

O,p-DDD[2,2-bis(parachlorophenyl)-1,1-dichloroethane]

O,p-DDD[2,2-bis(parachlorophenyl)-1,1-dichloroethane], which acts on adrenal glands, is used in the treatment of inoperable adrenal cortical carcinoma. In a series of 115 patients treated by Lubitz et al. (1973), neurological and/or muscular toxicity observed in 60% of cases was most frequent after gastrointestinal toxicity. The most frequent neurological symptoms and signs found in those patients were lethargy and somnolence, indicating cerebral dysfunction.

CEREBELLAR DYSFUNCTION

Signs of cerebellar dysfunction, mainly ataxia, have been observed following the administration of 5-FU, procarbazine, BCNU, and OpDDD, which cross the blood-brain barrier readily. Whereas it has been established that 5-FU may cause cerebellar lesions (Riehl and Brown, 1964), it is not quite certain that the ataxia observed in patients treated with procarbazine, BCNU, or OpDDD is caused by cerebellar injuries. Ataxia is also frequently present in children with leukoencephalopathies related to the treatment of CNS leukemia.

5-FU

Cerebellar dysfunction occurs in less than 1% of patients treated with 5-FU. It is characterized by ataxia, unsteadiness of gait, slurred and scanning speech, dysmetria, and coarse nystagmus. In addition to the four cases reported by Riehl and Brown in 1964, Moertel et al. (1964) observed 18 cases of cerebellar ataxia in 360 patients treated with 5-FU given as 9-day loading courses.

Cerebellar signs were also reported in patients receiving weekly intravenous doses of 15 to 20 mg/kg body weight (Horton et al., 1970; Bateman et al., 1971; Gottlieb and Luce, 1971; Gailani et al., 1972; Piro et al., 1972). In most cases, cerebellar signs induced by 5-FU are transitory and disappear after treatment is discontinued or with a change in schedule or doses of chemotherapy. Therefore, the pathological aspects of cerebellar lesions caused by 5-FU are poorly documented. Koenig and Patel (1970) tentatively attributed the cerebellar dysfunction of patients treated with 5-FU to depression of Krebs cycle by 5-FU catabolites.

Procarbazine

Like other forms of nervous toxicity, ataxia is more commonly seen when procarbazine is given intravenously; however, this route is not commonly used because of the neurotoxic side effects. Even when the drug is given orally, ataxia may be observed (Stolinsky et al., 1970), but it is rare, mild, and seldom a dose-limiting factor for drug administration.

BCNU and OpDDD

Dizziness, loss of equilibrium, and ataxia have been reported in 9.4% of 223 patients treated with intravenous BCNU, 1.5 mg/kg body weight/day for 5 days (Ramirez et al., 1972).

Ataxia was also observed in the same patients treated with OpDDD (Lubitz et al., 1973).

Differential Diagnosis

Toxic cerebellar effects of chemotherapy should be differentiated from cerebellar metastases and so-called carcinomatous cerebellar atrophy. Cerebellar metastases frequently produce symptoms and signs of intracranial hypertension that are lacking in toxic cerebellar dysfunction. However, nausea and vomiting attributable to chemotherapy may be present in patients with cerebellar dysfunction caused by chemotherapy. Signs of cerebellar metastases do not regress after discontinuation of chemotherapy but may be relieved by corticosteroids. Carcinomatous atrophy of the cerebellum (Chapter 8) is more difficult to differentiate from toxic lesions. These cerebellar diseases are rare and are seldom associated with digestive neoplasm where 5-FU is most commonly used.

INVOLVEMENT OF MENINGES, SPINAL CORD, OR NERVE ROOTS

The involvement of meninges, spinal cord, or nerve roots is present primarily in patients treated by intrathecal injections of MTX and/or ara-C. Recently, Gutin et al. (1976) have used intrathecal thio-tepa in the treatment of meningeal carcinomatosis and have observed a neurological toxicity limited to transient paresthesia of limbs. At present, however, intrathecal thio-tepa is not widely used.

Unlike the encephalopathies previously described, in patients treated for meningeal leukemia these neurological side effects begin immediately or shortly after the last intrathecal injection of the drug. They consist of chemical meningitis, which is fairly common, or spinal cord or root lesions, which occur infrequently.

Meningeal Syndrome

The meningeal syndrome is characterized by headaches, vomiting, nuchal rigidity, Kernig's sign, photophobia, delirium, and obtundation. A more or less complete and severe clinical manifestation of this chemical arachnoiditis occurs 2 to 4 hr after intrathecal injection of MTX. Meningism is rarely seen after a first administration of MTX but its frequency increases with the number of intrathecal injections. In most patients, signs of meningism appear within 72 hr. The incidence of the meningeal reaction attributable to intrathecal MTX varies considerably from one report to another: it was observed in 9.8% of children with meningeal leukemia treated by Sullivan et al. (1969), in 40% of 73 patients reported by Geiser et al. (1975) in 55% of patients treated by Duttera et al. (1972) for overt meningeal leukemia, and in 90% of 120 patients reported by Naiman et al. (1970).

CSF changes consisting of an increase of cells, mainly mononuclear, and a moderate increase of protein levels are seen not only in patients with clinical signs of meningism but also in cases without overt meningeal reaction. This chemical arachnoiditis is related to MTX concentrations in the CSF. Using low doses of MTX (10 μg/kg q. 2 to 3 days), Mollica et al. (1971) observed no neurological complications in 300 patients who received prophylactic CNS treatment. Furthermore, Bleyer et al. (1973) have shown that the neurotoxicity of intrathecal MTX was more frequent and more severe in cases where CSF-MTX concentrations were high. Those concentrations are not easily predictable when MTX is given by lumbar puncture. Concentrations of intrathecal MTX may be unexpectedly high in patients with overt meningeal leukemia, in which the transport of MTX from CSF to the systemic circulation may be impaired. This could explain a higher incidence of neurotoxic side effects after intrathecal MTX in patients receiving curative treatment as compared to those receiving prophylactic therapy. Other factors have also been considered in the pathogenesis of meningeal reaction after intrathecal injection of MTX: (1) The presence of chemical preservatives (methylhydroxybenzoate, propylhydroxybenzoate, benzyl alcohol), which are neurotoxic, could contribute to the side effects observed with intrathecal MTX; but chemical meningitis is not prevented by omission of preservatives (Naiman et al., 1970). (2) Injection of relatively large (±20 ml) volumes of water or saline, used as MTX solvents, to a poorly buffered medium, such as CSF, results in ionic changes which may cause some neurotoxic effects. In fact, the use of Elliot's B solution as MTX solvent markedly reduced the percentage of meningeal reactions (Duttera et al., 1972; Geiser et al., 1975).

Toxic effects of intrathecal MTX in CNS prophylaxis are less frequent in patients receiving concomitant cranial irradiation (Geiser et al., 1975) and may be reduced by the addition of dexamethazone to the intrathecal chemotherapy.

Ara-C is frequently used in both prophylactic and curative treatment of meningeal leukemia; its intrathecal injection produces headaches, vomiting, fever, and meningisms similar to those observed with MTX (Band et al., 1973).

Lesions of Spinal Cord and/or Nerve Roots

Paraparesis, paraplegia, quadriplegia, sensory changes, and bladder and intestinal paralysis, often preceded by radicular pain, have been occasionally reported after intrathecal administration of MTX (Table 4.4). Most of these patients were treated for overt meningeal leukemia; half recovered spontaneously, sometimes very rapidly. Pathological examinations performed in few cases showed demyelination of the nerve roots and/or white matter of the spinal cord (cases 1 and 8, Table 4.4). The involvement of the peripheral nervous system (PNS), at least in one of these patients, was demonstrated by the study of nerve conduction velocities (case 10, Table 4.4).

In the majority of these cases, neurological signs occurred immediately or within 24 hr after the intrathecal injection of MTX. Their pathogenesis remains obscure. In case 4 (Table 4.4), the same neurological deficit occurred after a lumbar puncture not followed by drug administration and after MTX or ara-C intrathecal injections. In case 8 (Table 4.4), the same neurological signs were produced by MTX and ara-C. These observations suggest that the lesions may not be related to the structure or to the mode of action of the drugs injected intrathecally.

LESIONS OF PERIPHERAL AND CRANIAL NERVES

Of the various anticancer drugs, the vinca alkaloids have the highest toxicity for the peripheral and cranial nerves. However, signs of usually mild peripheral neuropathy have been observed after the administration of procarbazine, 4-demethylepipodophyllotoxin-β-D ethylidene glucoside (VP 16–213), 5-azacytidine, cis-platinum, and OpDDD. In addition, optic neuritis has been reported in patients receiving BCNU, and retinal abnormalities were observed in some patients treated with CCNU.

Vinca Alkaloids

Four vinca alkaloids—VCR, vindesine, vinblastine, and formyl leurosine—are presently available for cancer chemotherapy. These substances block the cell metaphase by binding mitotic-spindle protein. They also prevent the formation of neurofilaments, disrupt those already formed, and impair the axoplasmic transport. The neurotoxicity of vinca alkaloids is attributed to these effects. However, the affinity for tubulin and microtubules, which appears to be the same for different vinca derivatives in *in vitro* experiments (Himes et al., 1976; Donoso et al., 1977), cannot account for the marked differences in clinical neurotoxicity of these drugs. Other factors, such as drug absorption, tissue distribution, or metabolism, are probably involved.

VCR

VCR is the most neurotoxic drug used in cancer chemotherapy; its clinical use is limited by neurological side effects. The severity of the peripheral neuropathy produced by VCR is dose related. It is usually heralded by paresthesia (tingling, burning, pinching, and numbness) in hands, feet, and perioral area. Ankle jerks disappear shortly after, followed by patelar reflexes and upper-limb tendon reflexes. Distal weakness starting in the lower limbs appears gradually, usually for total doses of more than 15 mg (Whitelaw et al., 1963; Hildebrand and Coërs, 1965; Slander et al., 1969; Holland et al., 1973). The onset of weakness should justify the discontinuation of treatment, since there is no specific therapy.

Cranial nerve lesions may be observed after VCR administration. The most commonly involved cranial nerves are the recurrent laryngeal nerve (Bohannon et al., 1963; Holland et al., 1973; Whittaker and Griffith, 1977), oculomotor nerves (ptosis without pupillary abnormalities or diplopia, Albert et al., 1967; Slander et al., 1969), and facial nerves (Slander et al., 1969).

The features of VCR neuropathy are quite symmetrical. Although mononeuropathies have been attributed to VCR (Levitt and Prager, 1975), in our opinion marked asymmetry in the distribution of neurological deficits is not consistent with the diagnosis of VCR neurotoxicity.

VCR-induced neuropathy is slowly reversible after drug discontinuation. The persistence of peripheral nerve lesions caused by VCR may be related to the lack of collateral regeneration of terminal axons demonstrated in muscle biopsy studies (Hildebrand and Coërs, 1965). Examination of muscle biopsies has also shown that a variable degree of peripheral neuropathy is present

TABLE 4.4. *Acute weakness after intrathecal MTX and ara-C*

References	Pat. No.	Intrathecal treatment			Clinical features	
		Drug	No. inject.	Dose (ma)	Onset after last LP	Symptoms and signs
Sullivan and Windmiller (1966)	1	MTX	20	100^a	24 hr	Paraplegia, T_6–T_8 sensory level
Back (1969)	2	MTX	13 (3 courses)	120^a	Immediate	Leg pain, leg rush, paraplegia, T^3 sensory level
Baashawe et al. (1969)	3	MTX	9	135^a	Immediate	Paraplegia and anesthesia of groin
	4	MTX	10	150^a	Immediate	Weakness and anesthesia of r. foot
		ara-C	2	82^a	Immediate	Pain in r. T_{2-10} plus weakness and anesthesia of r. foot
Pasquinucci et al. (1970)	5	MTX	53 (3 courses)	306^a	40 hr	Paralysis of legs, trunk, and neck, hypoesthesia of legs
Baum et al. (1971)	6	MTX	6	72^b	10 days	Weakness of 4 limbs and r. VII nerve
	7	MTX	5	60^b	12–24 hr	Flaccid paraplegia, depressed reflexes
Saiki et al. (1972)	8	MTX	5	95^a	12 hr	Bilateral T_{10} pain, paraplegia, bladder paralysis, T_{10} sensory level
		ara-C	1	20^a	Immediate	Leg pain, flaccid paraplegia
Bleyer et al. (1973)	9	MTX	6	90^b	Progressive after 4th injection	Facial and abdominal pain, bladder and intestinal ileus, quadriplegia
Luddy and Gilman (1973)	10	MTX	5	93^a	36 hr	Abdominal pain, flaccid paraplegia, and sensory level
Gemon et al. (1973)	11–18		1–60		30 min–24 hr (8 days in 1 case)	Primarily sensory deficit (2 cases), paraplegia (5 cases)
Meyer et al. (1976)	19	MTX	5	125^a	Immediate	Leg pain, flaccid quadriplegia, tendon reflexes abolished

Abbreviations: MTX, methotrexate; ara-C, cytosine arabinoside; LP, lumbar puncture; pat., patient; ^{a}, total dose; ^{b}, per square meter.

Evolution	Pathology
Death after 7 mo.	Demyelination myelomalacia plus perivascular infiltrate of CNS not given
Death after 30 min	—
Recovery within 2 hr	—
Recovery within 20 min	—
Recovery within 90 min	—
Started to improve after 48 hr	—
Improved partially	—
Spastic paraplegia	—
Reversible within 5 days	Demyelination of root and spinal cord white matter + perivascular infiltration
Death 1 mo. later	
Death 21 days after initiation of i.t. MTX	Residual leukemia
Paraplegia persisted for more than 33 mo.	—
Two deaths, 2 recoveries, 2 quadriplegia	—
Death after 2 hr	Blastic infiltration, thickening of meninges

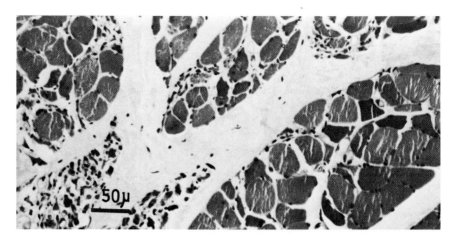

FIG. 4.1. Small and large group muscles atrophy pattern in the tibialis anticus in a patient with a severe peripheral neuropathy attributed to the combination of VCR and isoniazid.

in all patients treated with VCR; 50 to 80% of such patients will show clinical signs of polyneuritis. Nerve conduction velocity is either normal or abolished (Hildebrand and Coërs, 1965). Several factors, such as age, diabetes, preexisting neurological diseases, and other neurotoxic drugs may increase the sensitivity of the PNS to VCR. The incidence of neurotoxicity caused by VCR is three times greater in adults than in children (Whitelaw et al., 1963). An unusually severe neuropathy was observed by Weiden and Wright (1972) in a patient with Charcot-Marie-Tooth syndrome after only 4 mg VCR. Additive neurotoxicity of VCR and isoniazid or *l*-asparaginase,

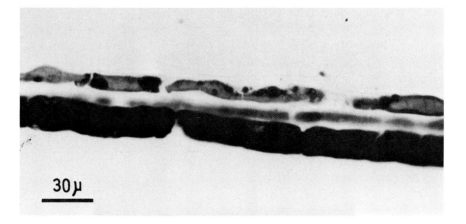

FIG. 4.2. Teased axons of sciatic nerve stained with osmium tetroxide showing various stages of axonal degeneration in a patient with a severe peripheral neuropathy attributed to the combination of VCR and isoniazid.

based on individual observations, was suggested by us (Figs. 4.1 and 4.2) (Hildebrand and Kenis, 1971, 1972), but these observations require further confirmation. VCR also produces dysfunction of the autonomic nervous system, resulting in constipation, ileus, urinary retention, and hypotension.

Constipation, accompanied by colicky abdominal pain, is seen in about one-third of patients treated with VCR. It occurs usually in the early course of the treatment. Adynamic ileus may follow constipation, and deaths have been attributed to this complication (Holland et al., 1973). The severity of constipation is not related to that of the peripheral neuropathy. Atonic bladder and urinary retention is a rare complication of VCR therapy (Slander et al., 1969; Gottlieb and Cuttner, 1971). Orthostatic hypotension has been reported in patients treated with VCR alone (Slander et al., 1969, Carmichael et al., 1970) or in combination with procarbazine (Aisner et al., 1974).

Other Vinca Alkaloids

Other vinca alkaloids are less neurotoxic than VCR. Vinblastine has been used for a long time, especially in the chemotherapy of lymphomas. Its side effects are mainly hematological, but mild peripheral neuropathies and cranial nerve lesions, such as vocal cord paralysis, have been reported (Brook and Schreiber, 1971). Clinical experience with formyl leurosine is very limited at present, but its neurotoxicity is probably mild.

Vindesine is also a new compound; it has an intermediate neurotoxicity between VCR and vinblastine. The neurotoxicity of vindesine is enhanced in patients previously treated with vincristine.

Procarbazine

Paresthesia and depression of deep tendon reflexes have been observed in 10% of patients treated with oral procarbazine by Brunner and Young (1965) and in 17% by Samuels et al. (1967). The peripheral neuropathy caused by procarbazine is mild and reversible.

VP 16–213

Peripheral neuritis was observed in six of 65 patients treated with VP 16–213, 300 to 400 mg/day for 5 days with a 9-day rest period between each (Falkson et al., 1975). The neurotoxicity, considered by the authors as drug related, is mild and reversible.

5-Azacytidine

Eight of 17 adult leukemic patients treated with intravenous 5-azacytidine, 200 to 250 mg/m^2/day for 5 days by Levi and Wiernik (1976), experienced a fairly severe neuromuscular toxicity (muscle tenderness and weakness) in addition to CNS side effects.

Cis-Platinum

Several cases of neurotoxicity have been reported in the *DCT Newsletter* (April, 1977). They consist of peripheral neuropathies of the upper and/or lower extremities (six cases) and seizures (four cases). Most of these reactions were observed in patients treated for periods longer than 6 months.

OpDDD

Peripheral neuropathy is mentioned by Lubitz et al. (1977) among neurotoxic side effects in some cases treated with OpDDD. Weakness was found in one-fifth of these 115 patients; however, the authors do not indicate whether this is due to neurological or muscular dysfunction.

Nitrosureas

Peripheral neuropathies were not reported in patients receiving nitrosureas, but optic neuritis was tentatively attributed to BCNU (McLennan, 1976), and retinal abnormalities were reported in four patients with malignant gliomas treated with CCNU and radiotherapy or BCNU alone (*FDA Newsletter,* January, 1977).

REFERENCES

Aisner, J., Weiss, H. D., Chang, P., and Wiernik, P. H. (1974): Orthostatic hypotension during combination chemotherapy with vincristine (NSC-67574). *Cancer Chemother. Rep.,* 58:927–930.

Albert, D. M., Wong, V. G., and Henderson, E. S. (1967): Ocular complications of vincristine therapy. *Arch. Ophthalmol.,* 78:709–713.

Ariel, I. M. (1961): Intra-arterial chemotherapy for metastatic cancer to the brain. *Am. J. Surg.,* 102:647–650.

Aur, R., Verzosa, M., Hustu, O., Simone, J., and Barker, L. (1975): Leukoencephalopathy during initial complete remission in children with acute lymphocytic leukemia receiving methotrexate. *AACR Abstr.,* p. 92.

Back, E. H. (1969): Death after intrathecal methotrexate. *Lancet,* ii:1005.

Bagshawe, K., Magrath, J. T., and Golding, P. R. (1969): Intrathecal methotrexate. *Lancet,* ii:1258.

Band, P. R., Holland, J. F., Bernard, J., Weil, M., Walker, M., and Rall, D. (1973): Treatment of central nervous system leukemia with intrathecal cytosine arabinoside. *Cancer,* 32:744–748.

Bateman, J. R., Pugh, R. P., Cassidy, F. R., Marshall, G. J., and Lowell, E. I. (1971): 5-Fluorouracil given once weekly: Comparison of intravenous and oral administration. *Cancer,* 28:907–913.

Baum, E. J., Koch, H. F., Corby, D. G., and Plunket, D. C. (1971): Intrathecal methotrexate. *Lancet,* i:649.

Bethlenfalvay, N. C., and Bergin, J. J. (1972): Severe cerebral toxicity after intravenous nitrogen mustard therapy. *Cancer,* 29:366–369.

Bleyer, W., Drake, J. C., and Chabner, B. A. (1973): Neurotoxicity and elevated cerebrospinal fluid methotrexate concentration in meningeal leukemia. *N. Engl. J. Med.,* 291:770–773.

Bohannon, R. A., Miller, D. G., and Diamond, H. D. (1963): Vincristine in the treatment of lymphomas and leukemias. *Cancer Res.,* 23:613–621.

Borns, P. F., and Rancier, L. F. (1974): Cerebral calcification in childhood leukemia mimicking Sturge-Weber syndrome. *Am. J. Roentgenol.,* 122:52–55.

Brook, J., and Schreiber, W. (1971): Vocal cord paralysis: A toxic reaction to vinblastine (NSC-49842) therapy. *Cancer Chemother. Rep.,* 55:591–593.

Brunner, K. W., and Young, C. W. (1965): A methylhydrazine derivative in Hodgkin's disease and other malignant neoplasms: Therapeutic and toxic effects studied in 51 patients. *Ann. Intern. Med.,* 63:69–86.

Carmichael, S. M., Eagleton, L., Ayers, C. R., and Mohler, D. (1970): Orthostatic hypotension during vincristine therapy. *Arch. Intern. Med.,* 126:290–293.

Chabner, B. A., Sponza, R., Hubbard, S., Canellos, G. P., Young, R. C., Shein, P. S., and DeVita, V. T. (1973): High-dose intermittent intravenous infusion of procarbazine (NSC-77213). *Cancer Chemother. Rep.,* 57:361–363.

Cliford, P., Oettgen, H. G., Beecher, J. L., Brown, F. P., Harries, J. R., and Lawes, W. E. (1963): Nitrogen mustard therapy with aortic occlusion in nasopharyngeal carcinoma. *Br. Med. J.,* 1:1256–1260.

Costa, G., Hreshchyshyn, M., and Holland, J. F. (1962): Initial clinical studies with vincristine. *Cancer Chemother. Rep.,* 24:39–44.

Creaven, P. J., Malicz, T. J., Brecher, M. L., Wang, J. J., and Freeman, A. I. (1977): Methotrexate levels in cerebrospinal fluid during simultaneous intraventricular and high dose intravenous administration. *AARC Abstr.,* p. 110.

DeConti, R. C. (1971): Procarbazine in the management of late Hodgkin's disease. *JAMA,* 215:927–930.

Donoso, J. A., Green, L. S., Heller-Bettinger, I. E., and Samson, F. E. (1977): Action of the vinca alkaloids vincristine, vinblastine, and desacetyl vinblastine amine on axonal fibrillar organelles in vitro. *Cancer Res.,* 37:1401–1407.

Duttera, M. J., Gallelli, J. F., Kleinman, L. M., Tangrea, J. A., and Wittgrove, A. C. (1972): Intrathecal methotrexate. *Lancet,* i:540.

Falkson, G., van Dyk, J. J., van Eden, E. B., van der Merve, van den Bergh, J. A., and Falkson, H. C. (1975): A clinical trial of the oral form of 4'-demethyl-epipodophyllotoxin-β-D ethylidene glucoside (NSC-141540) (VP 16–213). *Cancer,* 35:1141–1144.

Flament-Durand, J., Ketelbant-Balasse, P., Maurus, R., Regnier, R., and Spehl, M. (1975): Intracerebral calcifications appearing during the course of acute lymphocytic leukemia treated with methotrexate and X rays. *Cancer,* 35:319–325.

French, J. D., West, P. M., von Amerongen, F. K., and Magoun, W. H. (1952): Effects of intracarotid administration of nitrogen mustard on normal brain and brain tumors. *J. Neurosurg.,* 9:379–389.

Gailani, S., Holland, J. F., Falkson, G., Leone, L., Burningham, R., and Larsen, V. (1972): Comparison of treatment of metastatic gastrointestinal cancer with 5-fluorouracil (5-FU) to a combination of 5-FU with cytosine arabinoside. *Cancer,* 29:1308–1313.

Gams, R. A., and Carpenter, J. T. (1974): Central nervous system complications after combination treatment with adriamycin (NSC-123127) and 5-(3.3-dimethyl-1-triazeno) imidazole-4-carboxamide (NSC-45388). *Cancer Chemother. Rep.,* 58:753–754.

Geiser, C. F., Bishop, Y., Jaffe, N., Furman, L., Traggis, D., and Frei, E., III (1975): Adverse effects of intrathecal methotrexate in children with acute leukemia in remission. *Blood,* 45:189–194.

Gemon, M. F., Weil, M., Jacquillat, C., and Ambrosy, A. (1973): Accidents neurologiques du méthotrexate intra-rachidien. *Actual. Hematol.,* 7:22–25.

Gerner, R. E., Moore, G. E., and Didolkar, M. S. (1973): Chemotherapy of disseminated malignant melanoma with dimethyl-triazeno imidazole carboxamide (NSC-45388). *Cancer Chemother. Rep.,* 54:471–473.

Gottlieb, J. A., and Cuttner, J. (1971): Vincristine-induced bladder atony. *Cancer,* 28:674–675.

Gottlieb, J. A., and Luce, J. K. (1971): Cerebellar ataxia with weekly 5-fluorouracil administration. *Lancet*, i:138–139.

Green, A. A., and Naiman, J. L. (1968): Chlorambucil poisoning. *Am. J. Dis. Child.*, 116:190–191.

Greenwald, E. S. (1976): Organic mental changes with fluorouracil therapy. *JAMA*, 235:248–249.

Gutin, P. H., Weiss, H. D., Wiernik, P. H., and Walker, M. D. (1976): Intrathecal N,N',N''-triethylenethio-phosphoramide [thio-tepa (NSC-6396)] in the treatment of malignant meningeal disease. *Cancer*, 38:1471–1475.

Haskell, C. M., Canellos, G. P., Leventhal, B. G., Carbone, P. P., Block, J. B., Serpick, A. A., and Selawry, O. S. (1969a): L'asparaginase: Therapeutic and toxic effects in patients with neoplastic disease. *N. Engl. J. Med.*, 281:1028–1034.

Haskell, C. M., Canellos, G. P., Leventhal, B. G., Carbone, P. P., Serpick, A. A., and Hansen, H. H. (1969b): L-asparaginase toxicity. *Cancer Res.*, 29:974–975.

Hendin, B., DeVivo, D. C., Torack, R., Lell, M. E., Ragab, A. H., and Vietti, T. (1974): Parenchymatous degeneration of the central nervous system in childhood leukemia. *Cancer*, 33:468–482.

Hildebrand, J., and Cöers, C. (1965): Etude clinique, histologique et électrophysio-logique des neuropathies associées au traitement par la vincristine. *Eur. J. Cancer*, 1:51–58.

Hildebrand, J., and Kenis, Y. (1971): Additive toxicity of vincristine and other drugs for the peripheral nervous system. *Acta Neurol. Belg.*, 71:486–491.

Hildebrand, J., and Kenis, Y. (1972): Vincristine neurotoxicity. *N. Engl. J. Med.*, 287:517.

Himes, R. H., Kersey, R. N., Heller-Bettinger, I., and Samson, F. E. (1976): Action of the vinca alkaloids vincristine, vinblastine, and desacetyl vinblastine amide on microtubules in vitro. *Cancer Res.*, 36:3798–3802.

Holland, J. F., Scharlau, C., Gailani, S., Krant, M. J., Olson, K. B., Horton, J., Shnider, B. I., Lynch, J. J., Owens, A., Carbone, P. P., Colsky, J., Grob, D., Miller, S. P., and Hall, T. C. (1973): Vincristine treatment of advanced cancer: A cooperative study of 392 cases. *Cancer Res.*, 33:1258–1264.

Horton, J., Olson, K. B., Sullivan, J., Reilly, C., Shnider, B., and the Eastern Coopera-tive Oncology Group (1970): 5-Fluorouracil in cancer: An improved regimen. *Ann. Intern. Med.*, 73:897–900.

Jacquillat, C., Weil, M., Bussel, A., Loisel, J. P., Rouesse, T., Larrieu, M. J., Boiron, M., Dreyfus, B., and Bernard, J. (1970): Treatment of acute leukemia with 1-aspara-ginase. Preliminary results of 84 cases. In: *Experimental and Clinical Effects of L-Asparaginase*, edited by E. Grundmann and H. F. Oettgen, pp. 263–278. Springer-Verlag, Berlin.

Jean, R., Navarro, M., Marty, M., Dossa, D., Margueritte, G., Montoya, F., and Maury, M. (1976): Encéphalopathie aigüe au cours du traitement des lympho-blastoses de l'enfant. *Ann. Pediatr.*, 23:789–795.

Kay, H. E. M., Knapton, J. P., O'Sullivan, J. P., Wells, D. G., Harris, R. F., Innes, E. M., Stuart, J., Schwartz, F. C. M., and Thompson, E. N. (1972): Encephalopathy in acute leukaemia associated with methotrexate therapy. *Arch. Dis. Child.*, 47:344–354.

Kleinknecht, D., Jacquillat, C., Weil, M., Najean, Y., Tanzer, J., Boiron, M., and Bernard, J. (1967): Les accidents neurologiques centraux de la vincristine. *Nouv. Rev. Hematol. Fr.*, 7:132–136.

Koenig, H., and Patel, A. (1970): The acute cerebellar syndrome in 5-fluorouracil chemotherapy: A manifestation of fluoroacetate intoxication. *Neurology (Minneap.)*, 20:416.

Land, V. J., Sutow, W. W., Fernbach, D. J., Lane, D. M., and Williams, T. E. (1972): Toxicity of 1-asparaginase in children with advanced leukemia. *Cancer*, 30:339–347.

Levi, J. A., and Wiernik, P. H. (1976): A comparative clinical trial of 5-azacytidine and guanazole in previously treated adults with acute nonlymphocytic leukemia. *Cancer*, 38:36–41.

Levitt, L. P., and Prager, D. (1975): Mononeuropathy due to vincristine toxicity. *Neurology (Minneap.)*, 25:894–895.

Lôo, H., and Zittoun, R. (1969): Intoxication aigüe à forme comateuse par la vincristine. *Gaz. Med. Fr.*, 76:2693–2698.

Lubitz, J. A., Freeman, L., and Okun, R. (1973): Mitotane use in inoperable adrenal cortical carcinoma. *JAMA*, 223:1109–1112.

Luddy, R. E., and Gilman, P. A. (1973): Paraplegia following intrathecal methotrexate. *J. Pediatr.*, 83:988–992.

McIntosh, S., and Aspnes, G. T. (1973): Encephalopathy following CNS prophylaxis in childhood lymphoblastic leukemia. *Pediatrics*, 52:612–615.

McLennan, R. (1976): In a letter to Investigational Drug Branch, NCI, June, 1976.

Meadows, A. T., and Evans, E. E. (1976): Effects of chemotherapy on the central nervous system. *Cancer*, 37:1079–1085.

Meyer, R., Bergerat, J. P., Lang, J. M., and Oberling, F. (1976): Accident neurologique mortel après methotrexate intra-rachidien. *Nouv. Presse Med.*, 5:149.

Moertel, C. G., Reitemeier, R. J., Bolton, C. F., and Shorter, R. G. (1964): Cerebellar ataxia associated with fluorinated pyrimidine therapy. *Cancer Chemother. Rep.*, 41:15–18.

Mollica, F., Schiliro, G., Pavone, L., and Collica, F. (1971): Intrathecal methotrexate. *Lancet*, ii:771.

Moure, J. M. B., Whitecar, J. P., and Bodey, G. P. (1970): Electroencephalogram changes secondary to asparaginase. *Arch. Neurol.*, 23:365–368.

Naiman, J. N., Rupprecht, L. M., Tanyeri, G., and Philippidis, P. (1970): Intrathecal methotrexate. *Lancet*, i:571.

Norrell, H., Wilson, C. B., Slagel, D. E., and Clark, D. B. (1974): Leukoencephalopathy following the administration of methotrexate into the cerebrospinal fluid in the treatment of primary brain tumors. *Cancer*, 33:923–932.

Oettgen, H. F., Stephenson, P. A., Schwartz, M. K., Leeper, R. D., Tallal, L., Tan, C. C., Clarkson, B. D., Golbey, R. B., Krakoff, I. H., Karnofsky, D. A., Murphy, M. L., and Burchenal, J. H. (1970): Toxicity of E. coli l-asparaginase in man. *Cancer*, 25:253–278.

Ohnuma, T., Holland, J. F., Freeman, A., and Sinks, L. F. (1970): Biochemical and pharmacological studies with asparaginase in man. *Cancer Res.*, 30:2297–2305.

Owens, G., and Hatiboglu, I. (1961): Clinical evaluation of sodium thiosulfate as a systemic neutralizer of nitrogen mustard. *Ann. Surg.*, 154:895–897.

Pasquinucci, G., Pardini, R., and Fedi, F. (1970): Intrathecal methotrexate. *Lancet*, i:309.

Paterson, A. H. G., and McPherson, T. A. (1977): A possible neurologic complication of DTIC. *Cancer Treat. Rev.*, 61:105–106.

Piro, A. J., Wilson, R. E., Hall, T. C., Aliapoulios, M. A., Nivenny, H. B., and Moore, F. D. (1972): Toxicity studies of fluorouracil used with adrenalectomy in breast cancer. *Arch. Surg.*, 105:95–99.

Price, L. A., Goldie, J. H., and Hill, B. T. (1975): Methodichlorophen as antitumour drug. *Br. Med. J.*, 2:20–21.

Price, L. A., and Jamieson, P. A. (1975): The central nervous system in childhood leukemia. II. Subacute leukoencephalopathy. *Cancer*, 35:306–318.

Ramirez, G., Wilson, W., Grage, T., and Hill, G. (1972): Phase II evaluation of 1,3-bis(2-chloroethyl)-1-nitrosourea (BCNU, NSC-409962) in patients with solid tumors. *Cancer Chemother. Rep.*, 56:787–789.

Reitemeier, R. J., Moertel, C. G., and Blackburn, C. M. (1964): Vincristine (NSC-67574) therapy of adult patients with solid tumors. *Cancer Chemother. Rep.*, 34:21–23.

Riehl, J. L., and Brown, J. (1964): Acute cerebellar syndrome secondary to 5-fluorouracil therapy. *Neurology*, 14:254.

Rosemberg, S. (1974): Encéphalopathie apparue au cours d'un traitement par la vincristine. Observation anatomoclinique. *Arch. Fr. Pediatr.*, 31:391–398.

Rubinstein, L. J., Herman, M. M., Long, T. F., and Wilbur, J. R. (1975): Disseminated necrotizing leukoencephalopathy: A complication of treated central nervous system leukemia and lymphoma. *Cancer*, 35:291–305.

Saiki, J. H., Thompson, S., Smith, F., and Atkinson, R. (1972): Paraplegia following intrathecal chemotherapy. *Cancer*, 29:370–374.

Samuels, M. L., Leary, W. B., Alexanian, R., Howe, C. D., and Frei, E., III (1967): Clinical trials with N-isopropyl-α-(2 methylhydrazino)-p-tolnamide hydrochloride in malignant lymphoma and other disseminated neoplasms. *Cancer,* 20:1187–1194.

Schochet, S. S., Lampert, P. W., and Earle, K. M. (1968): Neurological changes induced by intrathecal sulfate. *J. Neurol. Exp. Neurol.,* 27:645–658.

Shapiro, W. R., Chernik, N. L., and Posner, J. B. (1973): Necrotizing encephalopathy following intraventricular instillation of methotrexate. *Arch. Neurol.,* 28:96–102.

Slander, S. G., Tobin, W., and Henderson, E. S. (1969): Vincristine-induced neuropathy: A clinical study of fifty leukemic patients. *Neurology (Minneap.),* 19:367–374.

Slater, L. M., Wainer, R. A., and Serpick, A. A. (1969): Vincristine neurotoxicity with hyponatremia. *Cancer,* 23:122–124.

Stolinsky, D. C., Solomon, J., Pugh, R. P., Stevens, A. R., Jacobs, E. M., Lowell, E. I., Wood, D. A., Steinfeld, J. L., and Bateman, J. R. (1970): Clinical experience with procarbazine in Hodgkin's disease, reticulum cell sarcoma, and lymphosarcoma. *Cancer,* 26:984–989.

Storti, E., and Quaglino, D. (1970): Dysmetabolic and neurological complications in leukemic patients treated with l-asparaginase. In: *Experimental and Clinical Effects of L-Asparaginase,* edited by E. Grundmann and H. F. Oettgen, pp. 344–349. Springer-Verlag, Berlin.

Sullivan, M. P., Vietti, T. J., Fernbach, D. J., Griffith, K. M., Yhaddy, T. B., and Watkins, W. L. (1969): Clinical investigations in the treatment of meningeal leukemia: Radiation therapy regimens versus conventional intrathecal methotrexate. *Blood,* 34:301–319.

Sullivan, M. P., and Windmiller, J. (1966): Side effects of amethopterin (methotrexate) administered intrathecally in the treatment of meningeal leukemia. *Med. Rec. Ann.,* 50:92–101.

Tashima, C. K. (1975): Immediate cerebral symptoms during rapid intravenous administration of cyclophosphamide (NSC-26271). *Cancer Chemother. Rep.,* 59:441–442.

Weiden, P. L., and Wright, S. E. (1972): Vincristine neurotoxicity. *N. Engl. J. Med* 286:1369–1370.

Weiss, H. D., Walker, M. D., and Wiernik, P. H. (1974): Neurotoxicity of commonly used antineoplastic agents (first part). *N. Engl. J. Med.,* 291:75–81.

Whitelaw, D. M., Cowan, D. H., Cassidy, F. R., and Patterson, T. A. (1963): Clinical experience with vincristine. *Cancer Chemother. Rep.,* 30:13–20.

Whittaker, J. A., and Griffith, I. P. (1977): Recurrent laryngeal nerve paralysis in patients receiving vincristine and vinblastine. *Br. Med. J.,* 1:1251–1252.

Whittaker, J. A., Parry, D. H., Bunch, C., and Weatherall, D. J. (1973): Coma associated with vincristine therapy. *Br. Med. J.,* 4:335–337.

Wolfson, S., and Olney, M. B. (1957): Accidental ingestion of a toxic dose of chlorambucil. *JAMA,* 165:239–240.

Chapter 5

Neurotoxicity of Radiation Therapy

Radiotherapy may injure both the central and the peripheral nervous systems (CNS and PNS). Toxic effects of irradiations, which occur early after the completion of radiotherapy, are usually transitory and mild. On the other hand, the late neurotoxicity of irradiations is severe and usually irreversible.

Radiotherapy may also lead to the development of nervous system lesions by enhancing the neurological side effects of certain drugs, either by an enhancement of toxicity or by increasing the permeability of the blood-brain barrier to neurotoxic substances. Unfortunately, information from the literature concerning the tolerance of the human CNS to combined treatments with radiation and chemotherapy does not supply quantitative data on dose-reduction factors (van der Kogel et al., 1976).

Various clinical forms of neurological disorders caused by radiation therapy are listed in Table 5.1. The neurotoxic effects that are considered in this chapter concern the common forms of radiotherapy: X-rays (200 KV), γ-rays (Co^{60}, Betatron, or linear accelerator), or highly accelerated electrons (Betatron, linear accelerator). Other types of radiation, such as proton-beam or neutron-beam, have been used in the treatment of acromegaly (Kjellberg

TABLE 5.1. *Neurological disorders caused by radiotherapy*

Early and Transitory Disorders
    Cerebral disorders
        In leukemic children with CNS prophylaxis
        In adults with brain tumors
    Myelopathies
        Lhermitte's sign

Late and Severe Disorders
    Cerebral lesions
        Secondary to thrombosis of neck vessels
        Late necrotic encephalopathy
    Myelopathies
        Acute myelopathy
        Lower motor neuron syndrome
        Chronic progressive myelopathy
    Lesions of peripheral nerves
        Cranial nerves
        Brachial plexus

Induction of tumors

et al., 1968; Lawrence et al., 1970) and malignant gliomas (Parker et al., 1976). Neurological complications, including vertigo, cranial nerve palsies, and visual alterations, have been observed after proton-beam therapy (Dawson and Dingman, 1970; Braunstein and Loriaux, 1971; Kjellberg and Kliman, 1971). In patients with malignant gliomas treated with neutron-beam, a coagulative necrosis causing severe encephalopathy is regularly found at autopsy, thus limiting the use of this treatment (Parker et al., 1976).

EARLY AND TRANSITORY EFFECTS OF RADIOTHERAPY ON THE NERVOUS SYSTEM

Cerebral Disorders

A transient neurological disorder characterized by somnolence of varying degree has been described by Freeman et al. (1973) in children with acute lymphoblastic leukemia after prophylactic cranial irradiation. Treatment consisted of 2,400 rads delivered to the midplane of the cranium in 20 doses given over 28 days. These children also received four intrathecal injections of methotrexate (MTX) (10 mg/m²) at weekly intervals during irradiation. Clinical symptoms included somnolence varying from mild drowsiness to prolonged periods of sleep reaching 20 hr a day. There was no evidence of increased intracranial pressure nor of focal neurological signs. The syndrome was observed in 22 (79%) of 28 treated children: it was mild and might have passed unrecognized in 11 (39%), and severe in another 11. The younger patients tended to have the more severe symptoms. The somnolence appeared between 24 and 56 days and lasted 10 to 38 days. Cerebrospinal fluid (CSF) changes were inconstant and consisted of elevation of protein or increased number of mononuclear cells. During the somnolent phase, the EEG showed irregular, often rhythmic, activities at 3 to 7 cycles/sec. The syndrome was reversible in all patients and was tentatively attributed to transient disturbance of myelination. No pathological examinations were obtained.

Transitory deterioration of neurological status was observed by Boldrey and Sheline (1966) during the period following radiation therapy in patients with intracranial tumors and was attributed to treatment. Adverse symptoms and signs, such as nausea, headaches, ataxia, and drowsiness, were observed mainly during the second month following the discontinuation of radiotherapy. Unlike the somnolence syndrome reported by Freeman et al. (1973), the symptoms observed by Boldrey and Sheline (1966) were less frequent in childhood and infancy than in adults; their observation is not isolated but the incidence of the syndrome, found in 50% of their patients, appears unusually high today. The use of steroids, which improves the syndrome, may have decreased its frequency.

Brain edema has also been observed after high single doses of radiotherapy, i.e., 1,000 rads, sometimes given to patients with brain metastases to shorten the time of treatment.

Transient Radiation Myelopathy

A mild and transient form of myelopathy consisting of subjective sensory symptoms has been described in 10 to 15% of patients, mainly during the third month following the completion of radiotherapy on the spinal cord. Its onset is often insidious, consisting of tingling or numbness of extremities. Lhermitte's sign, characterized by electrical discharge sensations down the spinal cord and limbs, produced by flexing the neck, is often observed in these patients. Objective neurological examinations remain normal. This form of radiation myelopathy undergoes spontaneous resolution within 3 to 4 months. Transient myelopathy has been tentatively attributed to demyelination, especially of the posterior spinal tracts; oligodendrocytes, which synthetize myelin, are the cells most sensitive to radiation in the nervous tissue. Also, Lhermitte's sign is frequent in multiple sclerosis, a demyelinating disease.

There is some disagreement concerning the prognostic value of Lhermitte's sign. Some authors (Bloomer and Hellman, 1975) state that it is not related to subsequent late myelopathy, whereas others (Fishman, 1975) support an opposite view. Lhermitte's sign, found in 62 of 592 patients (11%) treated at Stanford for Hodgkin disease, is considerably more frequent than late progressive myelopathy, found in only one patient in this series (Kaplan, 1972).

LATE AND SEVERE EFFECTS OF RADIOTHERAPY ON THE NERVOUS SYSTEM

Cerebral Lesions

Thrombosis of the Cervical Carotid Arteries

Radiation-related lesions of the cervical carotid arteries and large intracranial vessels are characterized by constriction of the vessels due to medial fibroblastic thickening and focal degeneration of the elastic membrane. Partial or total thrombosis may eventually occur.

The incidence of such lesions is not known, but clinical manifestations due to obstructive diseases related to radiations are rare. Eight cases published in the literature during the last 10 years are summarized in Table 5.2. All patients received at least 5,000 rads. Neurological symptoms occurred from a few months to more than 20 years after radiotherapy. Sudden hemiparesis, hemiplegia, and aphasia were the most commonly observed signs, and were frequently heralded by transient ischemic attacks.

TABLE 5.2. Cerebral disorders caused by postirradiation arterial occlusions

References	Age	Sex	Dose of radiations on the carotid (rads)	Delay after irradiation	Main clinical features and angiography	Pathology	Primary diseases
Dormody et al. (1967)	20	F	10,500	11 mo.	TIA followed by hemiplegia	Fibrosis and thickening of vessels. Endothelial proliferation	Pituitary insufficiency
Hayward (1972)	55	M	8,250	27 yr	TIA; carotid obstruction	Adventitial fibrosis fragmentation of elastic membrane	Hyperthyroidism
Glick (1972)	54	F	5,700	16 yr	TIA followed by bilateral paralysis	Thrombosis of 2 carotids by atheromatous material and fat-laden macrophages	Cancer of vocal cords
Kagan et al. (1971)	21	F	8,300	6 mo.	TIA, hemiparesis, and aphasia; narrowing of carotid artery at the siphon	Foam cells	Hodgkin disease
Conomy and Kellermeyer (1975)	27	F	7,200	11 mo.	Sudden hemiplegia and aphasia	Fibrosis and thickening of vessels	Hodgkin disease
Painter et al. (1975)	8	F	6,000	> 4 yr	Narrowing of internal carotid		Glioma of óptic chiasma
	7	F	5,000	5.5 yr	Seizures, papilledema, hemiparesis, stenosis of anterior and midcerebral arteries		Retinoblastoma
	29	M	6,800	23 yr	Sudden hemiparesis, occlusion of anterior and midcerebral arteries		Facial hemangioma

TIA, transient ischemic attacks.

Similar arterial lesions and clinical features were also observed in patients with facial hemangioma (Wright and Bresnan, 1976) and neurofibromatosis (Hilal et al., 1971) treated by radiotherapy. However, it is still uncertain whether these vascular lesions were related to radiation or to the underlying disease.

Necrotic Radiation Encephalopathy

The majority of patients with brain lesions attributed to radiation therapy were treated for intracranial tumors. For instance, in the survey of Raskind (1967), in 104 cases of CNS damage related to radiation therapy, there were 19 pituitary tumors, one craniopharyngioma, and 40 gliomas. In the vast majority of the remaining patients, with miscellaneous CNS lesions or extra-neural neoplasms, late spinal lesions developed. In the study by Kramer (1968) of 57 patients with brain necrosis attributed to radiation therapy, 31 had gliomas and seven had pituitary tumors. The differentiation between clinical signs and symptoms due to recurrent brain tumors and radionecrosis may be extremely difficult. The incidence of postradiation encephalopathy, therefore, cannot be accurately assessed. The incidence is obviously related to irradiation doses. As pointed out by J. Bouchard (*personal communication*), these complications develop mostly under two sets of circumstances: either large tumor doses delivered over a relatively short period (i.e., 3,000 to 5,000 rads in 2 to 3 weeks) or after repetition of moderate to large doses over a period of 1 year or more. The late radiation brain necrosis usually appears 1 to 3 years after the completion of radiation therapy, but extreme delays ranging from 3 months to more than 15 years have been reported (Kramer, 1968).

Clinical Features

The clinical features consist of a progressive onset of focal deficits, such as hemiparesis, aphasia, and hemianopsia, related to the location of brain damage. Seizures have also been observed. Stupor and coma eventually occur after a period of several weeks to several months. Unlike those in patients with recurring brain tumors, signs of intracranial hypertension are not usually seen in radiation encephalopathy. However, cases of postirradiation necrosis presenting as space-occupying lesions with headaches and bilateral papilledema have been reported (Diengdoh and Booth, 1976). The differential diagnosis between radiation necrosis and tumor recurrence may remain difficult even after the performance of complementary examinations. EEG usually shows slow focal waves, the radionuclide brain scan an increased (focal) uptake, the angiography an avascular mass, and the CAT scan an area of decreased absorption that may be enhanced by contrast medium.

Residual intellectual and mental disorders may be present in long-time survivors irradiated for brain tumors, especially in children. Partial disability or inability of self care were reported by Bloom et al. (1969) in four of 22 patients with medulloblastomas and by Bamford et al. (1976) in six of 30 cases. It is uncertain to what extent irradiations rather than the primary neoplastic disease are responsible for the observed disorders. In the experience of other authors, no single florid case of mental deficiency has been observed in long-term survivors.

Visual loss, pituitary insufficiency, and lesions of the hypothalamus have been reported in patients with radionecrosis involving the nervous structures of the sellar area. These complications have been described after radiotherapy in various pathological conditions: (a) patients with pituitary tumors and craniopharyngiomas (Rosengren, 1958; Crompton and Layton, 1961; Raskin, 1967; Kramer, 1968; Ghatak and White, 1969), (b) patients with a normal pituitary gland suffering from menstrual irregularities, essential hypertension, malignant exophthalmos, or prostatic or breast carcinoma (Buys and Kerns, 1957; Fuks et al., 1976), (c) patients with brain tumors not directly involving the hypothalamic pituitary region (Shalet et al., 1975), and (d) patients with neoplasms of ethmoid sinus, cavum, and other tumors of head and neck (Ross et al., 1957; Shukovsky and Fletcher, 1972). Loss of vision is particularly frequent in patients with sphenoid tumors treated with doses of more than 7,000 rads. Of 15 such patients followed for a period of at least 4 years, six have lost sight in one eye and three in both eyes (Shukovsky and Fletcher, 1972). The loss of vision was caused by three types of lesions. Macular and retinal degeneration, consisting of multiple hemorrhages, neo-vascularization, exudates, and retinal atrophy, occurred in seven eyes 2 to 3½ years after radiotherapy. Optic nerve atrophy causing progressive loss extending over several months was observed 4 to 5 years after the completion of irradiations. Thrombosis of the central retinal artery occurred in two patients in whom a sudden loss of vision developed 9 and 15 months after radiotherapy.

The most frequent feature of pituitary lesion is an impaired growth hormone secretion (Shalet et al., 1975, 1976). Apparently, growth hormone-secreting cells are the cells most sensitive to irradiations. Cases of postradiation pituitary drowism are rare but have been reported (Fuks et al., 1976).

Pathology

Histologically, radiation encephalopathy consists of areas of focal necrosis, which may be prominent in patients with a short latency period after irradiation, and areas of demyelination (Fig. 5.1) of deep cerebral or cerebellar structures, which are predominantly found in cases with a long "free interval" (De Reuck and vander Eecken, 1975). Radiation necrosis is often distributed in areas of vascular supply (Fig. 5.2), and vascular lesions are found almost invariably in the arteries supplying the injured areas. These findings indicate

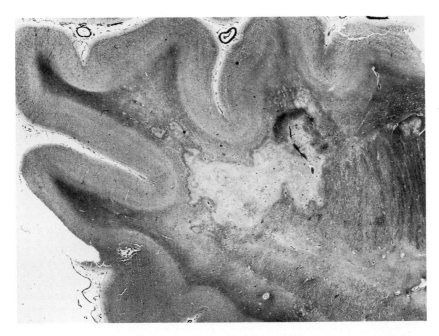

FIG. 5.1. Demyelination of the deep white matter in the right frontal lobe. The cortex and the arcuate fibers are spared. (Courtesy of Dr. H. vander Eecken.)

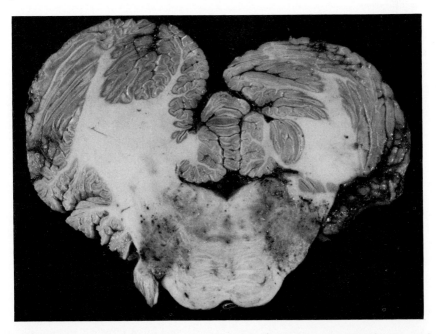

FIG. 5.2. Radiation necrosis of the lateral parts of the midpons (horizontal section, located in the supply area of the short circumferential branches of the brainstem). (Courtesy of Dr. H. vander Eecken.)

that the vascular changes are a major factor in the pathogenesis of radiation encephalopathy, but the role of a direct effect of irradiations on cerebral tissue must also be considered.

Treatment

The prognosis of radiation encephalopathy is poor; the majority of patients described died in the year following the onset of the disease. Immediate but transitory improvements may be achieved with corticosteroids (Martins et al., 1977). Long-term survivals and even apparent cures have been reported after surgical excision of the necrotic area. This treatment has been particularly successful in patients with extracranial tumors (Kramer, 1968; Takanchi et al., 1976).

Myelopathies

Three forms of late, usually irreversible, radiation myelopathy have been recognized: (1) acute myelopathy, (2) lower motor neuron syndrome, and (3) chronic progressive myelopathy.

Acute Myelopathy

Suddenly developing paraplegia or quadriplegia is especially observed in patients irradiated in the spinal cord area. This form of radiation myelopathy is believed to result from acute thrombosis of the spinal vessels because the onset of neurological signs is sudden.

Lower Motor Neuron Syndrome

Lower motor neuron syndrome is another very rare variety of radiation myelopathy; three cases were reported by Greenfield and Stark (1948) and a fourth by Sadowsky et al. (1976). The syndrome may, however, be more common than generally thought. We have recently observed two such cases, summarized in Table 5.3 together with the four previously reported patients. In addition, many cases of late myelopathy reported by Maier et al. (1969) in patients treated with radiation for testicular tumors probably belong in this category. The lower motor neuron syndrome appears 3½ to 23 months after the completion of radiotherapy. Neurological abnormalities are limited to the lower limbs in all cases thus far reported. They are characterized by muscle atrophy, weakness, depression of deep reflexes, and occasional fascicular twitchings. Objective sensory changes are absent. The disease is self-limiting after an evolution of several months. Patients' survival is considerably longer than in other forms of radiation myelopathies. The assumption that in this

TABLE 5.3. *Postradiation motor neuron syndrome*

References	Age	Sex	Radiotherapy (rads/days)	Delay of myelopathy (months)	Outcome (at publication)	Primary neoplasm
Greenfield and Stark (1948)	24	M	(a) 6,480/43 (b) 4,000/13	(a) 7 1/2 (b) 3 1/2	Alive	Adenoc. testis
	20	M	5,400/88	5	Alive	Teratoma testis
	28	M	5,488/82	4	Alive	Teratoid carcinoma testis
Sadowsky et al. (1976)	15	F	4,763/30	8	Alive	Medulloblastoma
Author's cases	45	M	6,200/3 frac- tioned doses (4½ yr)	23	Alive	Hodgkin disease
	27	F	4,000/29	3 1/2	Alive	Hodgkin disease

syndrome the motor spinal neurons are selectively injured has not been clearly demonstrated by pathological examination.

Chronic Progressive Myelopathy

Chronic progressive myelopathy is the most common form of late radiation myelopathy, with several hundred cases reported in the literature. Its incidence is difficult to assess. It was estimated by Palmer (1972) to occur in 2.9% of patients irradiated on the spine in a clinical series, and in 1.9% in patients in whom the diagnosis was confirmed by autopsy. These figures, however, are based only on publications reporting irradiation myelopathies and probably overestimate the actual incidence of the disease. For instance, in the Stanford series, late progressive myelopathy developed in only 0.15% (Kaplan, 1972).

The onset of the chronic progressive postirradiation myelopathy is delayed for several months to several years after completion of radiotherapy. The intervals observed for 83 patients in seven studies are given in Fig. 5.3; they vary from 3 to 50 months with a mean value of 13 and a median of 12 months.

Clinical Features

First symptoms consist of numbness and painful or burning paresthesias without precise radicular distribution, usually starting in the lower limbs. Many patients complain of inability to perceive pain or temperature. Motor deficits are seldom the initial sign of the disease; weakness appears first in

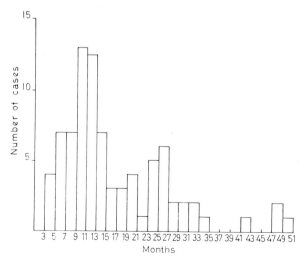

FIG. 5.3. Duration of the delay of the appearance of late progressive postirradiation myelopathy in 83 patients collected from seven clinical studies.

TABLE 5.4. Characteristics of progressive radiation myelopathy

| References | Number of PRM | Irradiations | | | | Main clinical features | Death | |
		Total irradiated patients	Dose (rads)	Duration (days)	Delay after irradiation (mo.)		After 6 mo.	After 1 yr
Boden (1948)	3 (small field) 3 (large field)	16 145	2,000 5,000 3,876–4,375	1 7 17	4–11 11–15	4 Spastic tri- or quadriplegia 2 Brown-Sequard syndrome	4	5
Dynes and Smedal (1960)	10	± 800	2,500–6,000	18–68	7–50	4 Paraplegia 3 Hemiplegia 3 Spasticity	2	4
Pallis et al. (1961)	5	—	4,410–8,700	28–42	7–18	2 Paraplegia 1 Quadriplegia 1 Brown-Sequard syndrome	—	—
Reagan et al. (1968)	10	1,018	4,000–6,900	10–56	5½–30	5 Paraparesis plus sensory loss 4 Brown-Sequard syndrome 1 Quadriparesis	3	5
Henry et al. (1971)	7	—	2,000–7,420	1–42	6–29	3 Paraparesis 3 Brown-Sequard syndrome 1 Quadriparesis	2	2
Jellinger and Sturm (1971)	12	—	1,455–9,700	19–61	3½–46	4 Paraplegia 4 Paraparesis 4 Brown-Sequard syndrome	9	11
Palmer (1972)	7	—	1,700–5,510	18–59	6–48	3 Weakness predominantly one side 3 Paraplegia or quadriplegia 1 Brown-Sequard syndrome	5	6
Combes et al. (1974)	27	—	4,000–13,400	18–75	6–48	9 Paraparesis or paraplegia 6 Quadriparesis or quadriplegia 6 Brown-Sequard syndrome 5 Hemiparesis or hemiplegia	—	—

the lower limbs, possibly followed by weakness of the upper limbs in patients with cervical lesions. Sensory levels and involvement of sphincters are commonly seen in patients with paraplegia or quadriplegia. As indicated in Table 5.4, a Brown-Sequard syndrome has been observed in about 25% of patients, but this usually represents a transitory stage eventually leading to paraplegia or quadriplegia. Hemiplegia has been observed in some cases (Table 5.4).

The prognosis for this form of radiation myelopathy is poor. The majority of patients will die within the year following the onset of neurological signs, infections of the urinary tract and bronchopneumonia being the most common causes of death.

Complementary Examinations

The CSF is usually normal although protein levels may be increased. This increase is slight (less than 100 mg/100 ml), but much higher values are found in rare cases where a block is seen on myelography. X-rays of the spine are normal. Myelography, usually normal, may show indentation of dye product, enlarged spinal cord with block, or spinal cord reduced in size.

The enlargement of the spinal cord is attributed to swelling. It may simulate an intramedullary tumor and has been repeatedly reported. (Palmer, 1972; Lechevalier et al., 1973; Marty and Minckler, 1973; Fogelholm et al., 1974). It is believed that spinal cord enlargement occurs early in the course of the disease.

Pathology and Pathogenesis

The majority of postirradiation spinal cord lesions are located at the cervical level. Histological studies show coagulative or hemorrhagic necrosis, which predominates in the white matter, mainly in the lateral and posterior spinal tracts; these may be replaced by eosinophilic material and fat-laden macrophages. Astroglial reaction is variable and may be poor. In the vicinity of the necrotic areas, myelin sheaths are swollen. Gray matter changes consist of rarefaction of neurons, especially in the anterior horns. Vessel alterations are constantly present, ranging from fibrinoid necrosis to hyalin thickening of vessel walls.

Telangiectasias, vessel obliterations, and fresh or organized thrombi are often observed. Vascular lesions are considered a major factor in the pathogenesis of late radiation myelopathy.

Although the majority of progressive radiation myelopathies have been observed in patients who received large doses of radiation, the most critical factor appears to be the daily dosage. Dose-time relationships of the tolerance of the spinal cord to irradiation was established by Boden in 1948 and reviewed by Pallis et al. in 1961. Although the observation of these criteria has decreased the incidence of radiation myelopathies, this complication has not disappeared and is still observed after administration of acceptable doses of radiotherapy. The overlapping of adjacent fields may be an important cause of the radiation myelopathies seen today.

Differential Diagnosis

The most common diagnostic error is to confuse radiation myelopathy with primary or metastatic intramedullary tumors. Clinical signs of radiation myelopathy and intramedullary tumors may be similar, especially in the initial phases. Myelography is more often normal in radiation myelopathy but, as mentioned previously, may simulate an intramedullary tumor.

Metastatic involvement of the epidural space is easier to distinguish from radiation myelopathy because radicular pain is almost invariably present, and abnormalities of X-rays of the spine and/or of myelography are found in more than 90% of patients with epidural space metastases.

Necrotizing carcinomatous myelopathy is a rare disease, first described by Mancall and Rosales (1964). This myelopathy has been found in association with different types of cancer, mainly lung carcinoma. Its onset and evolution are more rapid than those of late progressive radiation myelopathy.

Other spinal cord diseases, such as syringomyelia, multiple sclerosis, and nonspecific or syphilis vascular lesions, are sufficiently characteristic to allow distinction on the basis of clinical features. Amyotrophic lateral sclerosis is easy to distinguish from the lower motor neuron syndrome caused by radiation; the latter does not involve the upper limbs and is very rare.

Lesions of Peripheral Nerves

Lesions of peripheral nerves caused by radiation therapy have been observed primarily in two types of neoplastic diseases: (1) head and neck tumors, and (2) breast carcinomas.

Head and Neck Tumors

There were few examples of radiation damage to cranial nerves (Table 5.5) until the recent report by Berger and Bataini (1977) of 35 cranial nerve palsies which occurred in 25 patients treated over a 14-year period with high dose radiotherapy for head and neck tumors. Their observations suggest that the complication might in fact be more common than previously thought. As indicated in Table 5.5, the twelfth nerve is most frequently involved, followed by the tenth (recurrent laryngeal) and the eleventh nerves. The histological structure of the optic nerve differs from that of cranial and peripheral nerves. Their lesions caused by radiotherapy have been considered previously. Cranial nerve palsies, which occur after a long delay (12 to 100 months) and high dose irradiations (6,000 rads or more), must be differentiated from

TABLE 5.5. Cranial nerve lesions caused by radiation therapy

| References | No. of cases | Injured cranial nerves | Irradiations | | | Delay after irradiations (mo.) | Follow-up without evidence of cancer recurrence (yr) |
			Dose (rads)	Duration (days)			
Rider (1963)	1	Abduceus	550			1 (?)	—
Westbrook et al. (1974)	2	1 Recurrent laryngeal 1 Hypoglossal	7,500 8,500	44 50		30 98	7 10
Cheng and Shulz (1975)	4	4 Hypoglossal	6,000–8,000	30–48		36–106	1½–6
Berger and Bataini (1977)	25	19 Hypoglossal 9 Vagus 5 Spinal 1 Trigeminal	6,250–10,000	41–43		12–172	Over 1

lesions caused by metastases, which are a more common cause of cranial nerve paralysis. For instance, in the study by Westbrook et al. (1974), of 37 patients with breast cancer and vocal cord paralysis, the neurological lesion was caused by metastases in 32, by radiation fibrosis in two, and by other causes in three.

The differential diagnosis is based on the absence of other signs of tumor progression. Thus the length of the follow-up period and the quality of clinical investigations are critical when cranial nerve lesions are attributed to radiotherapy.

Breast Carcinomas

Radiation damage to brachial plexus and cranial nerve palsies occurs after a long delay, ranging from 6 months to more than 10 years. The vast majority of patients with radiation lesions of the brachial plexus are women treated for breast cancer (von Mumenthal, 1964; Stoll and Andrews, 1966; Maruyama et al., 1967; Steiner et al., 1971; Westling et al., 1972; Zenker et al., 1976). Typically, the first symptoms of the disease are sensory disturbances, such as numbness, paresthesia, radicular pain which may be quite severe, and hypoesthesia of the fingers. These symptoms are followed by motor signs. Both the lower and the upper part of the brachial plexus may be injured but complete involvement is infrequent. The incidence of radiation damage of the brachial plexus is related to the doses delivered, the duration of radiotherapy, and the dimensions of the irradiated fields (Westling et al., 1972). Thus in the report of Stoll and Andrews (1966), lesions of the brachial plexus attributed to radiotherapy were found in 73% of 33 women treated with 5,775 rads in 25 to 26 days and in 15% of 84 patients who received 5,100 rads in 25 to 28 days on supraclavicular and axillary areas. In the study of Westling et al. (1972), in 60% of patients treated with 5,400 ± 1,000 rads delivered in 23 days on large supraclavicular and axillary fields, plexus lesions developed, whereas this complication was not observed in women who received 4,400 ± 400 rads in 18 days. It appears from these observations that 5,000 rads given for 5 weeks or 4,500 rads for 20 days carry a low and acceptable risk of serious plexus lesions, especially if the fields of irradiations are not too large.

Histological examinations of radiation lesions of brachial plexus have revealed an intense fibrosis of connective tissues surrounding the nerve. Since peripheral nerves are among the most radioresistant tissues, postirradiation lesions of the nerve plexus are attributed to nerve constriction and interference with blood supply due to the fibrous tissue. Because vascular factors may be important, attempts to improve the neurological deficits of these patients by surgical decompression (Steiner et al., 1971) were not very successful. The differential diagnosis between plexus lesions due to neoplastic infiltration and radiotherapy is difficult, especially in patients with breast cancer in whom recurrence may be observed after a very long delay following the removal of the primary tumor. Radiation lesions tend to have a slower progression and involve the proximal segments of the upper limbs. They should also be considered in the absence of evidence of tumor progression elsewhere in the body.

INDUCTION OF TUMORS

Induction of malignant and benign tumors is a rare complication of radiation therapy. Kramer (1968) has summarized the eight individual cases of malignant tumors described 5 to 20 years after irradiation. All patients had pituitary adenomas and were treated by repeated courses of irradiation; all but two received high total doses. Six of these tumors were sarcomas (five fibrosarcomas) and two were anaplastic carcinomas. The role of irradiation in the genesis of brain tumors has been further confirmed by the survey conducted by Modan et al. (1974) in 11,000 children treated with low doses (350 to 400 rads/field) for ringworm. The group was followed for 12 to 23 years, and an abnormally high percentage of malignant and benign head and neck or brain tumors developed. The distribution of brain tumors was as follows: six definite and two probable malignant neoplasms, four meningiomas, one craniopharyngioma, and four benign tumors.

REFERENCES

Bamford, F. N., Morris Jones, P., Pearson, D., Ribeiro, G. G., Shalet, S. M., and Beardwell, C. G. (1976): Residual disabilities in children treated for intracranial space-occupying lesions. *Cancer,* 37:1149–1151.

Berger, P. S., and Bataini, J. P. (1977): Radiation-induced cranial nerve palsy. *Cancer,* 40:152–155.

Bloom, H. J., Wallace, E. N., and Henk, J. M. (1969): The treatment and prognosis of medulloblastoma in children. A study of 82 verified cases. *Am. J. Roentgenol.,* 105:43–62.

Bloomer, W. D., and Hellman, S. (1975): Normal tissue responses to radiation therapy. *N. Engl. J. Med.,* 293:80–82.

Boden, G. (1948): Radiation myelitis of the cervical spinal cord. *Br. J. Radiol.,* 249:464–469.

Boldrey, E., and Sheline, G. (1966): Delayed transitory clinical manifestations after radiotherapy treatment of intracranial tumors. *Acta Radiol.,* 5:5–10.

Braunstein, G. D., and Loriaux, D. L. (1971): Proton-beam therapy. *N. Engl. J. Med.,* 284:332–333.

Buys, N. S., and Kerns, T. C. (1957): Irradiation damage to the chiasm. *Am. J. Ophthalmol.,* 44:483–486.

Cheng, V. S. T., and Schulz, M. D. (1975): Unilateral hypoglossal nerve atrophy as a late complication of radiation therapy of head and neck carcinoma: A report of four cases and a review of the literature on peripheral and cranial nerve damages after radiation therapy. *Cancer,* 35:1537–1544.

Combes, P. F., Daly, N., Schlienger, M., and Humeau, M. (1974): Les myélopathies radiques tardives progressives. *J. Radiol.,* 56:815–825.

Conomy, J. P., and Kellermeyer, R. W. (1975): Delayed cerebrovascular consequences of therapeutic radiation. *Cancer,* 36:1702–1703.

Crompton, M. R., and Layton, D. P. (1961): Delayed radio necrosis of the brain following therapeutic X-radiation of the pituitary. *Brain,* 84:85–101.

Dawson, D., and Dingman, J. F. (1970): Hazards of proton-beam pituitary irradiation. *N. Engl. J. Med.,* 282:1434.

De Reuck, J., and vander Eecken, H. (1975): The anatomy of the late encephalopathy. *Eur. Neurol.,* 13:481–494.

Diengdoh, J. V., and Booth, A. E. (1976): Postirradiation necrosis of the temporal lobe presenting as a glioma. *J. Neurosurg.,* 44:731–734.

Dormody, W. R., Thomas, L. M., and Gurdjian, E. S. (1967): Postirradiation vascular insufficiency syndrome. Case report. *Neurology,* 17:1190–1192.

Dynes, J. B., and Smedal, M. I. (1960): Radiation myelitis. *Am. J. Roentgenol.,* 83: 78–87.

Fishman, R. A. (1975): Reactions to radiation therapy. *N. Engl. J. Med.,* 293:669–670.

Fogelholm, R., Haltia, M., and Anderson, L. C. (1974): Radiation myelopathy of cervical spinal cord simulating intra-medullary neoplasm. *J. Neurol. Neurosurg. Psychiatry,* 37:1177–1180.

Freeman, J. E., Johnston, P. G. B., and Voke, J. M. (1973): Somnolence after prophylactic cranial irradiation in children with acute lymphoblastic leukaemia. *Br. Med. J.,* 4:523–525.

Fuks, Z., Glatstein, E., Marsa, G. W., Bagshaw, M. A., and Kaplan, H. S. (1976): Long term effects of external radiotherapy on the pituitary and thyroid glands. *Cancer,* 37:1152–1161.

Ghatak, N. R., and White, B. E. (1969): Delayed radiation necrosis of the hypothalamus. *Arch. Neurol.,* 21:425–430.

Glick, B. (1972): Bilateral carotid occlusive disease following irradiation from carcinoma of the vocal cords. *Arch. Pathol.,* 93:352–355.

Greenfield, M. M., and Stark, F. M. (1948): Post-irradiation neuropathy. *Am. J. Roentgenol.,* 60:617–622.

Hayward, R. H. (1972): Arteriosclerosis induced by radiation. *Surg. Clin. North Am.,* 52:359–366.

Henry, P., Castaigns, G., Hoerni, B., and Touchard, J. (1971): La myélopathie progressive post-radiothérapeutique tardive. *J. Neurol. Sci.,* 14:325–340.

Hilal, S. K., Salomon, G. E., and Gold, A. P. (1971): Primary cerebral arterial occlusive disease in children. *Radiology,* 99:87–94.

Jellinger, K., and Sturm, K. W. (1971): Delayed radiation myelopathy in man. Report of twelve necropsy cases. *J. Neurol. Sci.,* 14:389–408.

Kagan, A. R., Bruce, D. W., and Di Chiro, G. (1971): Fatal foam cell arteritis of the brain after irradiation for Hodgkin's disease. Angiography and pathology. *Stroke,* 2:232–238.

Kaplan, H. S. (1972): *Hodgkin's Disease.* Harvard University Press, Cambridge, Mass.

Kjellberg, R. N., and Kliman, B. (1971): Proton-beam therapy. *N. Engl. J. Med.,* 284: 333.

Kjellberg, R. N., Shintain, A., Frantz, A. G., and Kliman, B. (1968): Proton beam therapy in acromegaly. *N. Engl. J. Med.,* 278:684–695.

Kramer, S. (1968): The hazards of therapeutic irradiation of the central nervous system. *Clin. Neurosurg.,* 15:301–318.

Lawrence, J. H., Tobias, C. A., Linfoot, J. A., Born, J. C., Lyman, J. T., Chong, C. Y., Manongain, E., and Wei, W. C. (1970): Successful treatment of acromegaly—Metabolic and clinical studies in 145 patients. *J. Clin. Endocrinol. Metab.,* 31:180–198.

Lechevalier, B., Humeau, F., and Hautteville, J. P. (1973): Myélopathies radiothérapiques "hypertrophiantes." *Rev. Neurol.,* 129:119–132.

Maier, J. G., Perry, R. H., Saylor, W., and Sulak, M. H. (1969): Radiation myelitis of the dorsolumbar spinal cord. *Radiology,* 93:153–160.

Mancall, E. L., and Rosales, R. K. (1964): Necrotizing myelopathy associated with visceral carcinoma. *Brain,* 87:639–656.

Martins, A. N., Johnston, J. S., Henry, J. M., Stoffel, T. J., and Di Chiro, G. (1977): Delayed radiation necrosis of the brain. *J. Neurosurg.,* 47:336–345.

Marty, R., and Minckler, D. S. (1973): Radiation myelitis simulating tumor. *Arch. Neurol.,* 29:352–354.

Maruyama, Y., Mylrea, M., and Logothetis, J. (1967): Neuropathy following irradiation. *Am. J. Roentgenol.,* 101:216–219.

Modan, B., Baidatz, D., Mart, H., Steinitz, R., and Levin, S. G. (1974): Radiation induced head and neck tumours. *Lancet,* i:277–279.

Painter, M. J., Chutorian, A. M., and Hilal, S. K. (1975): Cerebrovasculopathy following irradiation in childhood. *Neurology,* 25:189–194.

Pallis, C. A., Louis, S., and Morgan, R. L. (1961): Radiation myelopathy. *Brain,* 84: 460–479.

Palmer, J. J. (1972): Radiation myelopathy. *Brain,* 95:109–122.

Parker, R. G., Berry, H. C., Gerdes, A. J., Soronen, M. D., and Shaw, C. M. (1976): Fast neutron beam radiotherapy of glioma multiforme. *Am. J. Roentgenol.,* 127: 331–335.

Raskind, R. (1967): Central nervous system damage after radiation therapy. *Int. Surg.,* 48:430–441.

Reagan, T. J., Thomas, J. E., and Colby, M. Y., Jr. (1968): Chronic progressive radiation myelopathy. Its clinical aspects and differential diagnosis. *JAMA,* 203:106–110.

Rider, W. D. (1963): Radiation damage to the brain. A new syndrome. *J. Can. Assoc. Radiol.,* 14:67–69.

Rosengren, B. (1958): Two cases of atrophy of the optic nerve after previous roentgen treatment of the chiasmal region and the optic nerve. *Acta Ophthalmol.,* 36:874–877.

Ross, H. S., Rosenberg, S., and Fridmann, A. H. (1957): Delayed radiation necrosis of the optic nerve. *Am. J. Ophthalmol.,* 76:683–686.

Sadowsky, C. H., Sachs, E., and Ochoa, J. (1976): Postradiation motor neuron syndrome. *Arch. Neurol.,* 33:786–787.

Shalet, S. M., Beaurdwell, C. G., Morris-Jones, P. H., and Pearson, D. (1975): Pituitary function after treatment of intracranial tumours in children. *Lancet,* ii:104–111.

Shukovsky, L. J., and Fletcher, G. H. (1972): Retinal and optic nerve complication in high dose irradiation technique of ethmoid sinus and nasal cavity. *Radiology,* 104: 629–634.

Steiner, C., Fallet, G. H., Moody, J. F., Roth, G., Boussina, I., Maurice, P. A., Alberto, P., and Paunier, J. P. (1971): Lésions du plan brachial survenant après radiothérapie pour cancer du sein. *Schweiz. Med. Wochenschr.,* 101:1846–1848.

Stoll, B. A., and Andrews, J. T. (1966): Radiation-induced peripheral neuropathy. *Br. Med. J.,* 1:834–837.

Takenchi, J., Hanakita, J., Mitsynki, A., Abe, M., and Handa, H. (1976): Brain necrosis after repeated radiation therapy. *Surg. Neurol.,* 5:89–93.

van der Kogel, A. J., Van Bekkum, D. W., and Barendsen, G. W. (1976): Tolerance of CNS to total body irradiation combined with chemotherapy applied for the treatment of leukemia. *Eur. J. Cancer,* 12:1260–1263.

von Mumenthaler, M. (1964): Armplexusparesen im Anschluss on Röntgenbestrahlung. *Schweiz. Med. Wochenschr.,* 94:1070–1075.

Westbrook, K. C., Ballontyne, A. J., Eckler, N. E., and Brown, G. R. (1974): Breast cancer and vocal cord paralysis. *South. Med. J.,* 67:805–807.

Westling, P., Svensson, H., and Hele, P. (1972): Cervical plexus lesions following postoperative radiation therapy of mammary carcinoma. *Acta Radiol. Ther. (Stockh.),* 11:209–216.

Wright, T. L., and Bresnan, M. J. (1976): Radiation-induced cerebrovascular disease in children. *Neurology,* 26:540–543.

Zenker, R., Muller-Farber, J., and Fischer, R. (1976): Experience with limited mastectomy without postoperative irradiation in breast carcinoma. A preliminary report. *Med. Welt,* 27:470–471.

Chapter 6

Nervous System Infections in Patients with Cancer

Infections of the nervous system are rare in patients with cancer, accounting, in our experience (see Table 1 in the preface to this volume), for about 1% of neurological lesions. The 0.2% reported by Chernik et al. (1973) is even lower. However, it is important to recognize these complications because some may be successfully treated.

The distribution of microorganisms causing neurological infections in patients with cancer is quite different from that found in a general population. In fact, the agents of nervous system infections in cancer are similar to those found in other pathological conditions in which immunity is depressed (O'Loughlin, 1975), suggesting that immunodepression is an important factor in the pathogenesis of nervous system infections in patients with malignant tumors.

A second important factor predisposing patients with cancer to infections is neutropenia. The incidence of infections is significantly increased when the polymorphonuclear count is lower than 1,000 cells/mm^3, particularly under 500 cells/mm^3. Another predisposing circumstance for central nervous system (CNS) infection is head and spine surgery.

Most of the organisms causing infections in cancer patients are referred to as opportunistic. Generally, they are not pathogenic for hosts with a normal immune surveillance. Numerous mechanisms, such as intensive chemotherapy, prolonged administration of corticosteroids, irradiations, splenectomy (Eraklis and Filler, 1972), and destruction of the bone marrow by malignant cells, cause both neutropenia and depression of the immunological defense mechanism. In addition, immunodepression may be related to the neoplastic disease itself, particularly in patients with leukemia, lymphoma, and myeloma.

Table 6.1 gives the relative frequency of infections associated with neoplasms and indicates the main predisposing factors. Herpes zoster is by far the most common type of nervous system infection in cancer patients, followed by bacterial meningitis. Fungal meningites are comparatively less frequent and their incidence appears to decrease. Brain abscesses occur mainly after neurosurgery, and those due to fungi—mainly to *Aspergillus*—are becoming more frequent as the survival of immunodepressed patients with lymphoma increases. Finally, viral encephalitis and cerebral toxoplasmosis are rare and occur almost exclusively in patients with leukemias, lymphomas, and depressed immunological surveillance.

TABLE 6.1. Classification of nervous system infections in patients with cancer

Neurological infections	Relative frequency	Main associated neoplasms	Predisposing factors
Herpes zoster	Very frequent	Lymphoma, chronic lymphocytic leukemia, myeloma	Depressed cell immunity
Meningitis			
Bacterial	Frequent	Miscellaneous	Neutropenia, neurosurgery
Fungal (cryptococcus neoformans)	Fairly frequent (decreasing rate ?)	Lymphoma, leukemia	Depressed cell immunity
Abscesses			
Bacterial	Fairly frequent	Miscellaneous	Neutropenia, neurosurgery
Fungal (aspergillus)	Fairly frequent	Lymphoma, leukemia	Depressed cell immunity, pulmonary aspergillosis
Encephalitis			
Progressive multifocal leukoencephalopathy	Rare	Lymphoma, leukemia	Depressed cell immunity
Other viral encephalites	Very rare		
Toxoplasmosis	Rare		

HERPES ZOSTER

Herpes zoster is the most frequent infection of the nervous system in cancer patients. This viral infection injures primarily the posterior roots and the ganglia, in which hemorrhagic and inflammatory lesions are seen. In immunodepressed patients, Cowdry A inclusions are found in addition to inflammatory changes in ganglia cells, satellite cells, and fibroblasts (Fig. 6.1). These inclusions correspond to herpes virus particles (Fig. 6.2). The incidence of about 0.5% in the general population is markedly increased in patients with neoplastic diseases, particularly those with lymphomas, chronic lymphocytic leukemias, and myelomas. The highest incidence of herpes zoster was reported in Hodgkin disease, where it ranges from 9 to 25% (Wright and Winer, 1961; Casazza et al., 1966; Wilson et al., 1972; Feldman et al., 1973; Schimpff et al., 1972). In splenectomized patients with Hodgkin disease, Herpes zoster occurred in 24% and was the most frequent form of infection (Schimpff et al., 1975). However, the role of splenectomy as a predisposing factor remains controversial. Several factors, such as irradiation, chemotherapy, administration of corticosteroids, and advanced stages of Hodgkin disease, increase the incidence of Herpes zoster. The disease tends to develop in previously irradiated dermatomes.

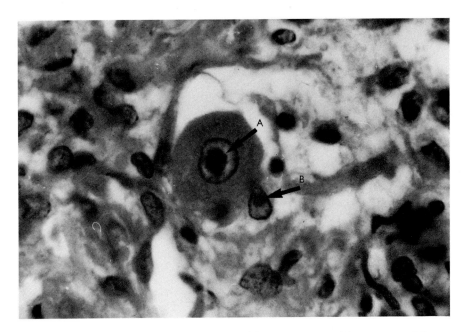

FIG. 6.1. Cowdry A inclusions in nuclei of ganglia cells (A) and satellite cells (B) in a trigeminal Herpes zoster in a patient with Hodgkin disease. (Courtesy of Dr. J. J. Vanderhaeghen.)

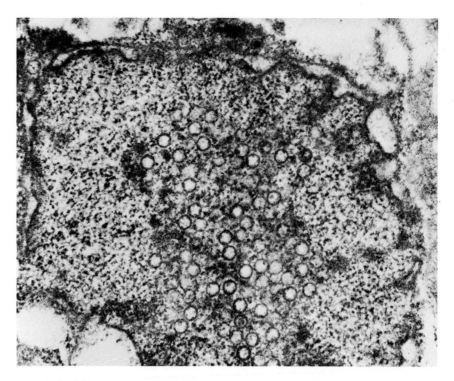

FIG. 6.2. Herpes virus particles demonstrated by electron microscope in root ganglia of leukemic patient with a generalized Herpes infection. (Courtesy of Dr. J. J. Vanderhaeghen.)

Clinical Signs

Herpes zoster is characterized by pain followed in the course of 3 to 4 days by papulovesicular skin lesions distributed in one or several sensory root territories. It is primarily an infection of spinal ganglia, but cranial nerves may also be affected (ophthalmic zoster and geniculate herpes). Weakness and subsequent muscle atrophy may appear, and a meningeal reaction may occur, causing lymphocytic pleocytosis and increase of protein in cerebrospinal fluid (CSF).

Herpes zoster virus is identical to the varicella virus, and disseminated infection (varicella zoster) may follow the localized disease, usually within a few days. Such a dissemination is rare, probably less than 1%, in a general population, but occurs more frequently in cancer patients because of chemotherapy, irradiation, and corticosteroids. In disseminated forms, death may occur (Merselis et al., 1964).

Treatment

It has been suggested that passive immunization with Herpes zoster immunoglobulin or plasma, if given early, might decrease the chances of dis-

semination of Herpes zoster in immunodepressed patients. This assumption is not supported by adequate clinical studies. It is recommended that the administration of chemotherapeutic agents and corticosteroids be discontinued when Herpes zoster develops in patients with cancer.

Even in immunodepressed patients, however, Herpes zoster usually heals spontaneously. Thus any therapeutic agent must have a high therapeutic (efficacy/toxicity) index. For this reason, the toxicity of iododeoxyuridine was judged unacceptable and the use of the drug restricted to topical application in Herpes keratitis.

In contrast, adenine arabinoside (ara-A) is extremely well tolerated, and its activity on pain, clearance of virus from vesicles, cessation of new vesicle formation, and time of pistulation have been shown in immunodepressed patients with Herpes zoster in a randomized cooperative study (Whitley et al., 1976). The drug is most effective when given during the first 6 days of the disease to younger patients (under 38 years of age) with a reticuloendothelial neoplasia.

MENINGITES AND MENINGOENCEPHALITES

After Herpes zoster, meningites and meningoencephalites are the most frequent forms of nervous system infections in patients with cancer. The majority of these infections are caused by bacteria that differ from agents responsible for meningitis in the general population. In addition, fungi account for a substantial percentage of meningites found in patients with malignant diseases.

Bacterial Meningites

When associated with cancer, bacterial meningites are most commonly seen in patients with severe neutropenia or impaired immunity, and after neurosurgical operations. The distribution of germs causing these infections is characterized by a high incidence of listeria monocytogenes, gram-negative bacilli, staphylococcus and various types of streptococcus. Pneumococcus is also frequently found and was responsible for 10 to 20 episodes of septicemia and meningitis observed in 18 of 200 children splenectomized for Hodgkin disease (Chilcote et al., 1976).

Meningococcus and Hemophilus influenzae, the most common germs found in general population meningitis, rarely cause meningeal infections in cancer patients.

Tuberculous meningitis is unusual in cancer patients, although tuberculosis is fairly common, especially in lung, head, and neck carcinomas and lymphomas (Kaplan et al., 1974). This complication has not developed in any of the 201 cancer patients with tuberculosis reported in Kaplan's study.

Exceptional cases of meningitis caused by Herpes simplex (Cappel and

Klastersky, 1973) or mumps (Rupprecht and Naiman, 1970) viruses have been reported in patients with acute leukemias.

Signs and CSF Changes

Clinically, bacterial meningites usually appears as acute pyogenic meningites characterized by the alteration of consciousness, signs of meningeal irritation, and general infection. Signs due to parenchymal lesions, such as seizures, fasciculations, or hemiplegia, are particularly frequent in infections due to Listeria monocytogenes (Buchner and Schneierson, 1968).

The CSF is under increased pressure, is usually cloudy, and contains large numbers of predominantly polymorphonuclear leukocytes. However, in patients with severe neutropenia, the CSF cellular reaction may be poor, in contrast with large quantities of bacilli found on CSF smear examination. Glucose CSF levels are frequently low and protein concentrations increased.

Treatment

In the treatment of gram-negative meningitis, potentially synergistic combinations of antibiotics, such as carbenicillin plus gentamicin, should be preferred to chloramphenicol. Nevertheless, the prognosis of these infections, treated systematically, is poor not only because infecting organisms are frequently resistant to a number of antiinfectious agents but also because most antibiotics fail to reach adequate concentration in the CSF. Therefore, intrathecal administration of gentamicin (10 mg every 24 hr) is advocated in patients with gram-negative meningitis. However, even high doses of gentamicin given by lumbar puncture may fail to eradicate meningeal infection, especially when ventriculitis develops. Intraventricular injection of both gentamicin and tobramycin yields more reliable and higher concentrations of antibiotics, especially in cisternal CSF, and appears more effective than treatments using the lumbar route.

Staphylococcal meningitis requires the administration of antistaphylococcal penicillins or vancomycin.

Listeria monocytogenes is susceptible to several antibiotics, generally at relatively low concentrations. Intravenous ampicillin appears to be the most effective and safe treatment of Listeria meningitis. Recovery from meningitis caused by Listeria monocytogenes seems to correlate best with CSF glucose concentrations; a concentration of less than 30 mg/100 ml is an unfavorable prognostic factor (Lavetter et al., 1971).

Fungal Meningites

In a series of 104 meningites observed in patients with cancer by Chernik et al. (1973), 31 were caused by fungi of which 28 were Cryptococcus neoformans. In a recent report, however, Chernik et al. (1977) observed a decrease in the percentage of cryptococcal meningitis at the Memorial Sloan-Kettering Cancer Center.

In cancer patients, nervous system infection by Cryptococcus neoformans is mainly associated with lymphomas (including Hodgkin disease) and chronic leukemias (Utz et al., 1975).

Signs and CSF Changes

The clinical picture of meningeal cryptococcosis is that of a subacute or chronic meningitis or meningoencephalitis. The onset is frequently insidious, sometimes mimicking primary psychiatric disorders (Martin et al., 1975); in rare cases, however, it may be sudden (Aberfeld and Gladstone, 1967). Headaches are the major presenting symptom. Meningeal symptoms usually predominate, but focal signs may be present. The main differential diagnoses of meningitis due to Cryptococcus neoformans are tuberculous and carcinomatous meningites. In all these conditions, CSF is usually clear, with low glucose and increased protein levels, and contains predominantly mononuclear cells. Cryptococcus neoformans may be demonstrated in CSF after India ink staining (without this procedure, the cryptococci may be mistaken for mononuclear cells) or by cultures on Sabouraud medium. However, the greatest diagnostic yield results from a search for both antigen and antibody in serum and CSF. A presumptive diagnosis of cryptococcal infection may be made in more than 90% of cases by this technique (Kaufman and Blumer, 1968).

Treatment

Satisfactory results in the treatment of cryptococcosis have been achieved with the combination of 5-fluorocytosine and amphotericin-B. Azotemia, thrombocytopenia, chills, and fever are frequent side effects of this treatment (Utz et al., 1975). According to Diamond and Bennet (1974), the presence of an underlying malignancy is an unfavorable factor for cure. Indeed, most of the poor prognostic factors, such as corticosteroid therapy, high CSF opening pressure, low CSF glucose, less than 20 leukocytes, presence of cryptococcus on CSF smear, isolation of cryptococcus from extraneural sites, and high titers of cryptococcal antigens in CSF and in serum, are found in patients with meningeal cryptococcosis and cancer.

ABSCESSES

Bacterial abscesses caused by a variety of organisms, mainly *Staphylococcus aureus,* Streptococcus, *Escherichia coli,* Pseudomonas, and bacteroids, are about equally distributed among patients with leukemias, lymphomas, head and spine surgery, and other neoplasms (Chernik et al., 1973). They may rarely develop within brain tumors. In the pituitary gland, this association was found in eight of 29 cases of pituitary abscesses reviewed by Dominique and Wilson (1977). Fungal abscesses are less frequent. They are found mainly in patients with lymphoma or leukemia and are due primarily to *Aspergillus* (Gruhn and Samson, 1963; Chernik et al., 1973, 1977; Meyer et al., 1973), less frequently to mucormycosis, and very rarely to *Candida albicans* or *Nocardia*. Fungal abscesses are usually associated with lung infections by the fungus.

An exceptional case of brain abscess caused by amoeba has been reported in a patient with Hodgkin disease (Jager and Stamm, 1972).

Signs and CSF Changes

The signs of brain abscess are basically those of intracranial space-occupying lesions. Signs of infections are mainly due to the extraneural focus which gave rise to brain abscess and may disappear when the primary focus is no longer active. Brain abscesses are multiple in about 50% of patients, and their differential diagnosis with brain metastases in patients with neoplasms is difficult and often requires surgery. Without craniotomy, the diagnosis of a large number of brain abscesses is made at necropsy.

The greatest danger of brain abscess may not be the infection but the mass effect. Lumbar puncture is therefore hazardous, yielding, in addition, only suggestive information (Samson and Clark, 1973). The changes of CSF are mainly related to the presence or absence of meningitis. When meningitis is absent, the CSF changes are those of an expanding cerebral lesion: increased intracranial pressure, moderate elevation of protein, usually normal glucose levels, and aseptic meningeal cellular reaction.

Treatment

The ideal treatment of brain abscesses is a total surgical removal of the abscess combined with antibiotics in full therapeutic doses. *Aspergillus* infections require the administration of amphotericin-B.

ENCEPHALITES

Encephalites are the less common forms of CNS infection in cancer patients. They are seen primarily in immunodepressed individuals with leukemia or lymphoma. Encephalites are caused by viral agents. *Toxoplasma gondii,* a protozoan organism, is a rare cause of encephalitis in cancer.

Progressive Multifocal Leukoencephalopathy

Aström et al. (1958) gave the name progressive multifocal leukoencephalopathy (PML) to a new form of encephalopathy they observed in two leukemic patients and one with Hodgkin disease. The disease is rare but not exceptional; in 1965, Vanderhaeghen and Perier reviewed 43 patients, including two personal cases, and Castaigne et al. (1974) were able to find 124 cases in the world literature.

Signs and CSF Changes

In the review of Vanderhaeghen and Perier (1965), 28 cases of PML (65%) occurred in patients with neoplastic diseases, mainly chronic lymphocytic leukemia (eight cases) and Hodgkin disease (eight cases). In patients without cancer, the underlying disease was usually a chronic and debilitating condition, such as sarcoidosis or tuberculosis. Only in rare cases is there no evidence of a predisposing disease (Fermaglich et al., 1970; Bolton and Rozdilsky, 1971).

The first signs of PML are mood changes and mental disorders. Focal neurological deficits are observed next, usually consisting of paresis, abnormalities of visual fields, and aphasia. Focal signs are unilateral in the beginning but rapidly become bilateral. Ataxia and difficulties of gait are present in about 25% of cases. Lesions of the cranial nerves and spinal cord are rare. Death occurs within a few months; 1 year survivals are very rare. However, long-time survivals of 5 (Hedley-Whyte et al., 1966), 10 (Kepes et al., 1976), and 19 years (Stam, 1966) have been observed, and exceptionally spontaneous remissions may occur (Hedley-Whyte et al., 1966). Complementary examinations are of limited value in the diagnosis of PML. The EEG shows diffuse, often asymmetrical slow waves. The composition of the CSF is usually normal, but moderately increased levels of protein or of the number of cells were observed.

Treatment

Few patients with PML were treated with antiviral agents such as 5-iodo-2'-deoxyuridine (IUDR) or cytosine arabinoside (ara-C). The observed therapeutic results are contradictory (Holden et al., 1971; Tarsy et al., 1973; Bauer et al., 1973), and better controlled trials are necessary.

Pathology and Pathogenesis

PML pathological changes consist of multiple, often confluent areas of demyelination in various parts of the CNS, including cerebellum (Fig. 6.3). Giant astrocytes are frequently seen in the center of the lesion but are not pathognomonic (Fig. 6.4). The most characteristic elements of these lesions are cells located at the demyelination edge (Fig. 6.5). These cells are characterized by large, homogenous, amphophilic nuclei and contain virions arranged in pseudocristalin formations, suggesting papovaviral particles (Zu

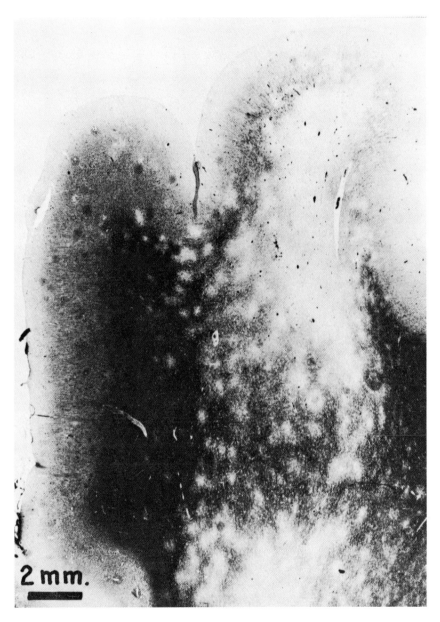

FIG. 6.3. Confluent areas of demyelination in case of progressive multifocal leukoencephalopathy. (Courtesy of Dr. J. J. Vanderhaeghen.)

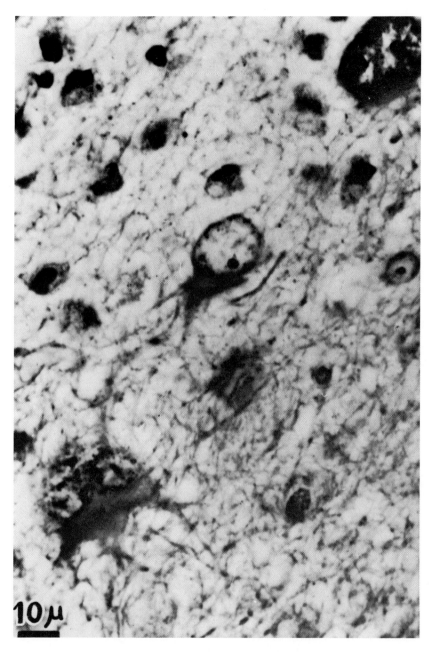

FIG. 6.4. Giant hypertrophic astrocytes present in the center of demyelinated areas in progressive multifocal leukoencephalopathy. (Courtesy of Dr. J. J. Vanderhaeghen.)

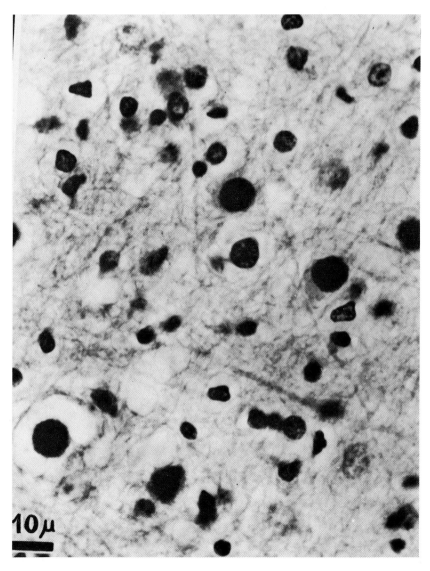

FIG. 6.5. Large homogenous amphophilic cells containing nuclei found at the edge of demyelination areas. (Courtesy of Dr. J. J. Vanderhaeghen.)

Rhein and Chou, 1965). Since 1965, this observation has been repeatedly confirmed (see Fig. 7.1). Further identifications of papovavirus in brain of patients with PML have been achieved more recently through fluorescent-antibody staining and electron microscopic agglutination techniques (Openda Narayan et al., 1973). In the last study, a JC type of papovavirus was identified in 11 of 13 cases studied. Papovaviruses are considered the causal agents

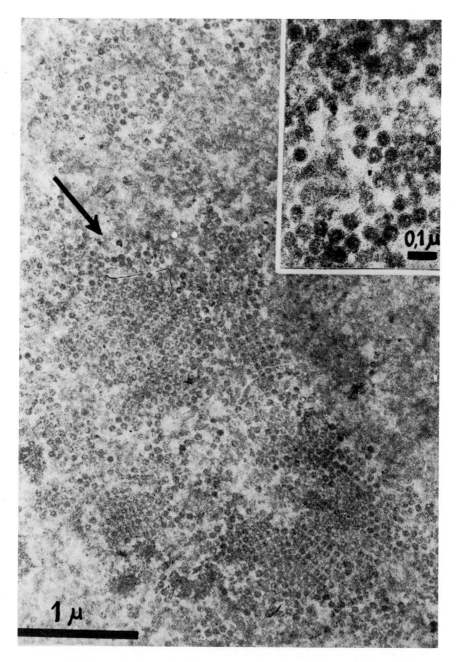

FIG. 6.6. Rounded viral particles, locally arranged in pseudocristalin formations shown by electron microscopy. (Courtesy of Dr. J. J. Vanderhaeghen.)

of PML, and this encephalitis is the first example of an association of viruses with a subacute or chronic human demyelinating disease. Since papovavirus may be oncogenic in laboratory animals, it is interesting to mention the association of glial brain tumor with PML observed by Castaigne et al. (1974).

Other Viral Encephalites

Encephalites caused by Herpes zoster-varicella, Herpes simplex, or measle virus are occasionally seen in cancer patients with an impaired immunity (Dayan et al., 1967; Chernik et al., 1973, 1977; Breitfeld et al., 1973; Feldman et al., 1975; Haltia et al., 1977). They occur mainly in leukemias and lymphomas, even during remission (Simone et al., 1972). With the exception of varicella virus encephalitis (the incidence of which varies considerably from one report to another) (Feldman and Cox, 1976), these infections are very rare and the number of reported cases does not clearly indicate that they actually occur more frequently in cancer patients. It is interesting to note that Herpes simplex encephalitis may have in anergic patients with lymphoma an atypical, slowly progressive course (Price et al., 1973).

In the carcinomatous polioencephalopathy, the presence of astroglial nodules and of lymphocytic infiltrations (see Figs. 8.1 and 8.2) suggests a viral etiology which has not yet been demonstrated.

Treatment

The therapeutic value of antiviral drugs, such as ara-A, ara-C, or iodo-deoxyceridine, has not been unequivocally established in viral encephalitis; it was even disproven in certain adequately controlled studies. In immunodepressed patients who had contact with varicella, the administration of zoster immunoglobulin or plasma is an effective means to prevent infection (Gershon et al., 1974; Feldman and Cox, 1976) when given within 3 days after exposure. The benefit of this passive immunization should be given to all immunodepressed varicella contacts.

Toxoplasmosis

Toxoplasmosis is the name given to infections by *Toxoplasma gondii*. This protozoan organism has a predilection for eyes and the CNS, which may be infected *in utero* (congenital forms) or during childhood or adult life. The acquired forms of CNS toxoplasmosis are seen almost exclusively in patients with impaired immunity, primarily in patients with malignant tumors. The types of neoplasms most frequently associated with toxoplasma encephalitis are chronic leukemias and lymphomas, mainly Hodgkin disease (Bernard et al., 1962; Cheever et al., 1965; Vietzke et al., 1968; Barlotta et al., 1969; de Crousaz and de Tribolet, 1972; Carey et al., 1973).

Signs and CSF Changes

The most common clinical features of acquired toxoplasma encephalitis are headaches, vomiting, drowsiness, disorientation, and coma. Focal signs, such as hemiparesis and jacksonian seizures, are present in about 50% of cases. Isotopic brain scan and angiography may demonstrate mass lesions. EEG abnormalities usually predominate in one hemisphere. CSF proteins are generally increased, but pleocytosis is inconstant and usually lower than 10 cells/mm^3. Toxoplasma antibody titers are increased in CSF and in serum.

Treatment

Despite treatment with sulfonamides (sulfamethazine, sulfapyrazine, or sulfadiazine) in combination with pyrimethamine, death, occurring within a few weeks, is the usual outcome, especially in patients with an underlying neoplasm.

Pathology

Pathological examination demonstrates multifocal necrotic lesions containing protozoan organisms, predominantly located in the gray matter. Astrocytic glial reaction and mainly perivascular lymphocytic infiltrations are found in areas of brain surrounding the necrotic foci. Small granulomas formed by epitheloid cells, lymphocytes, polymorphonuclear leukocytes, and glial cells frequently associated with pseudocysts containing *Toxoplasma gondii* are usually found in acquired toxoplasmosis, whereas massive calcifications, which are common in congenital forms, are not seen in adults with cerebral toxoplasmosis (Ghatak et al., 1970).

REFERENCES

Aberfeld, D. C., and Gladstone, J. L. (1967): Cryptococcol meningoencephalitis presenting like hemiplegia of sudden onset. *JAMA,* 202:1150–1151.

Alström, K. E., Mancall, E. L., and Richardson, E. P., Jr. (1958): Progressive multifocal leukoencephalopathy in hitherto unrecognized complication of chronic leukemic and Hodgkin's disease. *Brain,* 81:93–111.

Barlotta, F. M., Ochoa, M., Jr., Neu, H. C., and Ultmann, J. E. (1969): Toxoplasmosis, lymphoma, or both? *Ann. Intern. Med.,* 70:517–528.

Bauer, W. R., Turel, A. P., Jr., and Johnson, K. P. (1973): Progressive multifocal leukoencephalopathy and cytaraine. Remission with treatment. *JAMA,* 226:174–176.

Bernard, J., Boiron, M., Levy, J. P., Ripault, J., and Desmonts, G. (1962): Toxoplasmose généralisée associée à une leucémie aiguë. *Nouv. Rev. Fr. Hematol.,* 2:910–914.

Bolton, C. F., and Rozdilsky, B. (1971): Primary progressive multifocal leukoencephalopathy. *Neurology (Minneap.),* 21:72–77.

Breitfeld, V., Hashida, Y., Sherman, F. E., Odagin, K., and Yunis, E. J. (1973): Fatal measles infection in children with leukemia. *Lab. Invest.,* 28:279–291.

Buchner, L. H., and Schneierson, S. S. (1968): Clinical and laboratory aspects of listeria monocytogenes infections. With a report of ten cases. *Am. J. Med.,* 45:904–921.

Cappel, R., and Klastersky, J. (1973): Herpetic meningitis (type 1) in a case of acute leukemia. *Arch. Neurol.,* 28:415–416.

Carey, R. M., Kimball, A. C., Armstrong, D., and Lieberman, P. H. (1973): Toxoplasmosis clinical experiences in a cancer hospital. *Am. J. Med.,* 54:30–38.

Casazza, A. R., Duval, C. P., and Carbone, P. P. (1966): Summary of infectious complications occurring in patients with Hodgkin's disease. *Cancer Res.,* 26:1290–1296.

Castaigne, P., Rondot, P., Escourolle, R., Ribadeau-Dumas, J. C., Cathala, F., and Hauw, J. J. (1974): Leucoencephalopathie multifocale progressive et "gliomes" multiples. *Rev. Neurol.,* 130:379–392.

Cheever, A. W., Valsamis, M. P., and Robson, A. S. (1965): Necrotizing toxoplasmosis encephalitis and herpetic pneumonia complicating treated Hodgkin's disease. *N. Engl. J. Med.,* 272:26–29.

Chernik, N. L., Armstrong, D., and Posner, J. B. (1973): Central nervous system infections in patients with cancer. *Medicine,* 52:563–581.

Chernik, N. L., Armstrong, D., and Posner, J. B. (1977): Central nervous system infections in patients with cancer. Changing patterns. *Cancer,* 40:268–274.

Chilcote, R. R., Bachner, R. L., and Hammond, D. (1976): Septicemia and meningitis in children splenectomized for Hodgkin's disease. *N. Engl. J. Med.,* 295:798–800.

Dayan, A. D., Bhatti, I., and Gostling, J. V. T. (1967): Encephalitis due to herpes simplex in a patient with treated carcinoma of the uterus. *Neurology,* 17:609–613.

Diamond, R. D., and Bennett, J. E. (1974): Prognostic factors in cryptococcol meningitis. A study in 111 cases. *Ann. Intern. Med.,* 80:176–181.

de Crousaz, G., and de Tribolet, N. (1972): 1. Lymphogranulome de Hodgkin stabilisé et encéphalite nécrosante à toxoplasme. *Arch. Suis. Neurol. Neurochir. Psychiatry,* 110:1–12.

Dominique, J. N., and Wilson, C. B. (1977): Pituitary abscesses. Report of seven cases and review of the literature. *J. Neurosurg.,* 46:601–608.

Eraklis, A. J., and Filler, R. M. (1972): Splenectomy in childhood. A review of 1413 cases. *J. Pediatr. Surg.,* 7:382–388.

Feldman, S., and Cox, F. (1976): Viral infections and haematological malignancies. *Clin. Haematol.,* 5:311–328.

Feldman, S., Hughes, W. T., and Kim, H. Y. (1973): Herpes zoster in children with cancer. *Am. J. Dis. Child.,* 126:178–184.

Feldman, S., Hughes, W. T., and Kim, H. Y. (1975): Varicella in children with cancer: 77 cases. *Pediatrics,* 56:388–397.

Fermaglich, J., Hardman, J. M., and Earle, K. M. (1970): Spontaneous progressive multifocal leukoencephalopathy. *Neurology (Minneap.),* 20:479–484.

Gershon, A. A., Steinberg, S., and Brunell, P. A. (1974): Zoster immune globulin. A further assessment. *N. Engl. J. Med.,* 290:243–245.

Ghatak, N. R., Poon, T. P., and Zimmerman, H. M. (1970): Toxoplasmosis of the central nervous system in the adult. *Arch. Pathol.,* 89:337–348.

Gruhn, J. G., and Samson, J. (1963): Mycotic infections in leukemic patients at autopsy. *Cancer,* 16:61–73.

Haltia, M., Paetau, A., Vaheri, A., Erkkilä, H., Donner, M., Kaakinen, K., and Holmström, T. (1977): Fatal measles encephalopathy with retinopathy during cytotoxic chemotherapy. *J. Neurol. Sci.,* 32:323–330.

Hedley-Whyte, T. E., Smith, B. P., Tyler, H. R., and Peterson, W. P. (1966): Multifocal leukoencephalopathy with remission and five year survival. *J. Neuropathol. Exp. Neurol.,* 25:107–116.

Holden, E. M., Tarsy, D., Calabressi, P., and Feldman, R. G. (1971): Use of 5-iodo-2'-deoxyuridine in progressive multifocal leukoencephalopathy. *Neurology,* 21:448.

Jager, B. V., and Stamm, W. P. (1972): Brain abscesses caused by free-living amoeba probably of the genus Hartmannella in a patient with Hodgkin's disease. *Lancet,* ii: 1343–1345.

Kaplan, M. H., Armstrong, D., and Rosen, P. (1974): Tuberculosis complicating neoplastic disease: A review of 201 cases. *Cancer,* 33:850–858.

Kaufman, L., and Blumer, S. (1968): Value and interpretation of neurological tests for the diagnosis of cryptococcosis. *Appl. Microbiol.,* 16:1907–1912.

Kepes, J. J., Chou, S. M., and Price, L. W. (1976): Progressive multifocal leukoencephalopathy with 10-year survival in a patient with nontropical sprue. *Neurology,* 25:1006–1012.

Lavetter, A., Leedom, J. H., Mathies, A. W., Ivler, D., and Wehrle, P. F. (1971): Meningitis due to listeria monocytogenes. *N. Engl. J. Med.,* 285:598–603.

Martin, R. A., Bates, D., and Shaw, D. A. (1975): Cryptococcol meningoencephalitis. *Br. Med. J.,* 3:75–76.

Merselis, J. G., Jr., Kaye, D., and Hook, E. W. (1964): Desseminated herpes zoster. A report of 17 cases. *Arch. Intern. Med.,* 113:679–690.

Meyer, R. D., Young, L. S., Armstrong, D., and Yu, B. (1973): Aspergillosis complicating neoplastic disease. *Am. J. Med.,* 54:6–15.

O'Loughlin, J. M. (1975): Infections in the immunosuppressed patient. *Med. Clin. North Am.,* 59:495–501.

Openda Narayan, D. V. M., Penney, J. B., Jr., Johnson, R. T., Herndon, R. M., and Weiner, L. P. (1973): Etiology of progressive multifocal leukoencephalopathy. Identification of papovavirus. *N. Engl. J. Med.,* 289:1278–1282.

Price, R., Chernik, N. L., Horta-Barbara, L., and Posner, J. B. (1973): Herpes simplex encephalitis in an anergic patient. *Am. J. Med.,* 54:222–228.

Rupprecht, L. M. T., and Naiman, J. L. (1970): Meningitis due to mumps virus in a child with acute leukemia. *Pediatrics,* 46:942–945.

Samson, D. S., and Clark, K. (1973): A current review of brain abscess. *Am. J. Med.,* 54:201–210.

Schimpff, S. C., O'Connell, M. J., Greene, W. K., and Wiernik, P. H. (1975): Infections in 92 splenectomized patients with Hodgkin's disease. A clinical review. *Am. J. Med.,* 59:695–701.

Schimpff, S., Serpick, A., Stoler, B., Rumack, B., Mellin, H., Joseph, J. M., and Block, J. (1972): Varicella-zoster infection in patients with cancer. *Ann. Intern. Med.,* 76:241–254.

Simone, J. V., Holland, E., and Johnson, W. (1972): Fatalities during remission of childhood leukemia. *Blood,* 39:759–769.

Stam, F. C. (1966): Multifocal leukoencephalopathy with slow progression and very long survival. *Psychiatr. Neurol. Neurochir.,* 69:453–459.

Tarsy, D., Holden, E. M., Segarra, J. M., Calabresi, P., and Feldman, R. G. (1973): 5-Iodo-2'-deoxyuridine (IUDR; NSC-39661) given intraventricularly in the treatment of progressive multifocale leukoencephalopathy. *Cancer Chemother. Rep.,* 57:73–78.

Utz, J. P., Garriques, I. L., Sande, M. A., Warner, J. F., Mandell, G. L., McGehee, R. F., Duma, R. J., and Smith, S. (1975): Therapy of cryptococcosis with a combination of flucytosine and amphotericin B. *J. Infect. Dis.,* 132:368–373.

Vanderhaeghen, J. J., and Perier, O. (1965): Leuco-encephalite multifocale progressive. Mise en évidence de particules virales par la microscopie électronique. *Acta Neurol. Psychiatr. Belg.,* 65:816–837.

Vietzke, M. V., Golderman, A. H., Grimley, P. M., and Valsamis, M. P. (1968): Toxoplasmosis complicating malignancy. Experience at the National Cancer Institute. *Cancer,* 21:816–827.

Whitley, R. J., Ch'ien, L. T., Dolin, R., Galasso, G. J., Alford, C. A., Jr., and the Collaborative Study Group (1976): Adenine arabinoside therapy of herpes zoster in the immunosuppressed. NIAID collaborative antiviral study. *N. Engl. J. Med.,* 294:1193–1199.

Wilson, J. F., Marsa, G. W., and Johnson, R. E. (1972): Herpes zoster in Hodgkin's disease. Clinical, histologic and immunologic correlations. *Cancer,* 29:461–465.

Wright, E. T., and Winer, L. H. (1961): Herpes zoster and malignancy. *Arch. Dermatol.,* 84:242–244.

Zu Rhein, G. M., and Chou, M. (1965): Particles resembling paporava viruses in human cerebral demyelinating disease. *Science,* 148:1477–1479.

Chapter 7

Vascular and Hemostatic Disorders

The vast majority of cerebrovascular lesions seen in cancer patients are not directly related to the neoplastic disease. The neurological disorders discussed in this chapter, which occur in response to cardiac or vascular lesions or hematological disorders, are not seen exclusively in patients with cancer, but their incidence is increased in malignant diseases. Cardiac myxoma, which is histologically benign but may have a malignant clinical course, particularly because of its cerebral complications, is also considered.

EMBOLISMS

The most common sources of cerebral embolisms in a general population are atrial thrombi in patients with a high risk of fibrillation, cardiac mural thrombi due to recent infarctions, and mitral valve lesions. In patients with cancer, cerebral embolisms also suggest less common sources, such as nonbacterial thrombotic endocarditis, cardiac tumors, or lipid embolizations following lymphography.

Nonbacterial Thrombotic Endocarditis

Nonbacterial thrombotic endocarditis (NBTE), also called marantic endocarditis, degenerative verucal endocarditis, or terminal endocarditis, is found in large autopsy series in about 1% of patients, the figures ranging from 0.4 to 2.4% (Table 7.1). NBTE is seen mainly in debilitated, cachectic, and elderly patients. There are, however, frequent exceptions; 16 of 75 patients with NBTE reported by Rosen and Armstrong (1973) were described as obese, and the disease may affect young patients (Weinstein and Schlesinger, 1974). Malignant tumors, particularly mucin-secreting carcinomas, are the most frequent underlying disease. Tumors most commonly associated with NBTE are located in the digestive tract (mainly the stomach), lung, prostate, or female genital tract. Their distribution varies from one series to another (Table 7.1). The proportion of patients with NBTE who have an underlying malignant disease also varies from one study to another and is related to the type of hospital population.

TABLE 7.1. Distribution of underlying diseases in patients with NBTE

				Neoplasms								
References	Type of patient population	Autopsies (no.)	Patients with NBTE (incidence)	Digestive tract and annexes	Lungs, bronchus, larynx	Urinary tract	Genital tract and prostate	Breast	Lymphomas	Others	Total	Other diseases
MacDonald and Robbins (1957)	General	18,486	78 (0.4)	18	4	—	—	1	2	2	27	51
Barron et al. (1960)	General	3,054	33 (1.1)	11	10	1	4	—	—	2	28	5
Bryan (1969)	General	13,000	22 (of 43)	9	5	2	3	—	—	3	22[a]	0
Rosen and Armstrong (1973)	Cancer	7,840	75 (1.2)	13	18	8	13	14	6	3	75[a]	0
Chino et al. (1975)	General	3,404	80 (2.4)	31	6	11		—	—	2	50	30

[a] Only patients with confirmed malignant tumors and NBTE were selected.

Clinical Features

General Signs

The general signs of NBTE may be similar to those of infective endocarditis; leukocytosis and petechiae are frequently seen, and even fever is common. Heart murmur, usually transient, soft, systolic, and most prominent at left sternal border, is found in less than one-half of the cases. The most characteristic clinical expressions of NBTE are multiple infarctions of organs, primarily of brain, spleen, kidney, and heart. Another prominent feature is the association with intravascular coagulation (Reagan and Okazaki, 1974), which accounts for the high rate of venous and arterial thromboses and thrombocytopenia seen in NBTE. In patients with mucus-producing carcinoma, abnormal coagulation has been related to the activation of factor X by the mucus or to the liberation of tissue thromboplastic factors.

Neurological Signs

Neurological signs are the most prominent manifestations of NBTE not only because emboli are more often located in the brain than in any other organ but also because infarctions in other tissues produce clinical symptoms less frequently. Thus in the series of 78 patients reported by MacDonald and Robbins (1957), emboli arose in 11, of whom seven had brain lesions contributing to death. Ten of 33 cases with NBTE described by Barron et al. (1960) had cerebral lesions; these 10 cases accounted for 9.5% of the total cerebral embolisms observed by these authors. In 75 cases reported by Rosen and Armstrong (1973), large cerebral vessel emboli were found in 14 patients. Embolus size is larger in NBTE than in infective endocarditis, and large cerebral vessels are therefore preferentially obstructed. For instance, the midcerebral artery was occluded in 11 of 14 cases reported by Rosen and Armstrong (1973) and in six of 10 cases described by Barron et al. (1960). The majority of neurological manifestations of NBTE, such as seizures or focal neurological deficits, result from cardiogenic emboli and appear in the sudden and dramatic manner of cerebral embolisms. The terminal stroke, however, may be preceded by one or more episodes of neurological dysfunction, which may clear partially or completely. In other patients, the onset of neurological signs will be progressive (Reagan and Okazaki, 1974). In many patients, signs of diffuse cerebral dysfunction are present either alone or in association with focal deficits, suggesting the presence of smaller multiple vascular occlusions.

Cardiogenic emboli, however, are not the only cause of nervous system lesions in patients with NBTE. Intravascular coagulation, often associated with NBTE, may independently produce cerebrovascular occlusions (Reagan and Okazaki, 1974). In addition, the lowering of platelet levels due to intravascular coagulation contributes to subdural, subarachnoid, and cerebral hemorrhages. Finally, brain metastases may occur in patients with NBTE and a malignant disease.

The prognosis for cancer patients with neurological manifestations due to NBTE is very poor. The 10 cases reported by Barron et al. (1960) rarely survived longer than 2 months, and all patients described by Reagan and Okazaki (1974) died within 120 days of their first neurological manifestations. Any benefit of anticoagulants has not been demonstrated.

Pathology

NBTE lesions are located predominantly at aortic and mitral valves (Fig. 7.1). Varrucal material contains no polymorphonuclear leukocytes, round

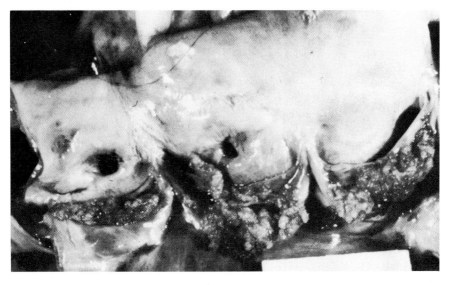

FIG. 7.1. Aortic valves bearing soft friable vegetations at the contact side of the leaflets. The patient has lung carcinoma and NBTE. (Courtesy of Dr. B. vanden Heule.)

cells, or Anitschkow cells characteristic of infective endocarditis. NBTE vegetations consist of amorphous acellular material composed of a mixture of platelets and fibrin (Fig. 7.2). A similar material was identified in the emboli occluding large cerebral vessels.

Cardiac Myxoma

Cardiac tumors are found in only about 0.05% of routine autopsies. Approximately one-half of them are myxomas. Cardiac myxomas are pediculated, almost always solitary tumors located preferentially in the left atrium near the fossa ovalis. Sarcomas, which occur next in frequency to myxomas,

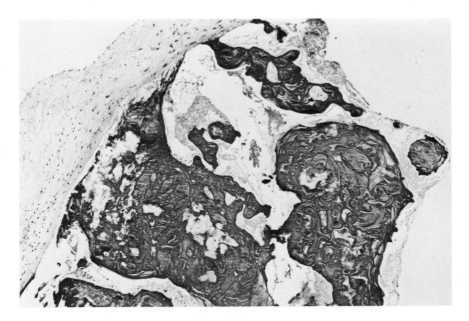

FIG. 7.2. Vegetation consisting of poorly cellular fibrinoid material loosely attached to a cardiac valve. The patient had lung carcinoma and NBTE. (Courtesy of Dr. B. vanden Heule.)

occur more frequently in the right side of the heart. Cardiac sarcomas may metastasize in the brain but do not produce embolizations.

Clinical Features

General Signs

The vast majority of cardiac myxomas are diagnosed in patients aged from 30 to 60 years. As in infective endocarditis and NBTE, fever, increased leukocytosis, increased erythrocyte sedimentation rate, anemia, and skin petechiae are frequently found (Greenwood, 1968). Cardiac murmurs, which are systolic or diastolic, or both, vary in time and with patient's position. Emboli, which occur in slightly less than one-half of patients with atrial myxoma, involve the brain, spleen, kidneys, retina, and skin. The tumor may also become symptomatic by obstructing cardiac flow and producing dyspnea, pulmonary hypertension, and pulmonary edema.

Neurological Signs

Clinical neurological manifestations are due to the obstruction of blood flow or embolisms (Schwartz et al., 1972; Yufe et al., 1976). Outflow obstruction produces syncopes and may cause occasional sudden deaths, whereas embolisms produce transient ischemic attacks, strokes, and seizures. Myelomalacia may develop after obstruction of spinal vessels (Wolman and Bradshaw, 1967). Embolization may be produced by fragments of tumor or blood clots that cover the surface of the tumor. The diagnosis of cardiac myxoma may be suggested on cerebral angiography by the presence of multiple aneurysms and irregular cerebral vessel fillings (Stoane et al., 1966; Burton and Johnston, 1970; Price et al., 1970; Damasio et al., 1975). Neurological deficits may also be due to subsequent growing of the myxomatous metastatic material from the cerebral vessels. The elevation of cerebrospinal fluid (CSF) protein in patients with myxoma brain emboli may be related to the growth of myxoma in the brain.

Treatment

Cardiac myxomas are histologically benign but clinically malignant, and are fatal if unrecognized and untreated. Diagnosis may be made by echocardiography, a reliable and innocuous diagnostic procedure. Definitive cure is achieved by surgical removal; recurrence does not usually occur, even without resection of the atrial wall underlying the tumor.

Postlymphographic Embolization

Lymphography is used routinely for staging of patients with lymphomas and other neoplasms, especially those of the pelvis, to determine the extent of metastatic lesions. Cerebral embolisms following this diagnostic procedure are rare. This neurological complication has been reviewed recently by Andersen et al. (1977), who added one personal observation to the 17 previously published cases. Eight of these 18 patients had lymphomas (six Hodgkin disease), five had other neoplasms, and five were investigated for nonneoplastic diseases.

Neurological symptoms and signs appeared immediately after lymphography in three cases. In most patients, the delay was of a few hours; the longest lasted 8 hr. Neurological features are those of diffuse cerebral dysfunction. Confusion, depressed responsiveness, stupor, lethargy, and coma were observed in eight patients. An akinetic mutism-like state developed in six others; and two had rigidity. Cortical blindness was seen in two patients and conus syndrome in one.

The outcome of postlymphographic embolism is usually favorable. Full recovery occurred in 13 cases within a few days to a few weeks. Three patients died: one from hematemesis, and another from possible electrolyte imbalance; psychotic signs persisted in one patient 6 months after lymphography.

There was histological proof of brain lipid embolism in only two cases. In others, the diagnosis was based on the evidence of retinal embolism, the presence of contrast medium on skull X-rays or elsewhere in the body, or opacification of renal parenchyma. Cerebral embolisms following lymphography, which occur after a much shorter latency than traumatic lipid embolisms, are attributed to direct obstruction of cerebral vessels by the contrast material. Two mechanisms may explain postlymphographic lipid embolisms: abnormal right-to-left shunts and passage of contrast medium through normal pulmonary capillaries. This passage is favored by lipid overloading of the lungs with contrast material. In addition, increased jugular pressure may favor the appearance of clinical manifestations of lipid emboli by enhancing cerebral edema (Andersen et al., 1977).

INTRACRANIAL BLEEDING

Thrombocytopenia, vasculitis caused by septicemia and high leukocytosis, metastases, and intravascular coagulation contribute to the increased incidence of intracranial hemorrhages in patients with cancer. These factors are most frequently present either alone or in combination in leukemic patients in whom intracranial bleeding is very frequent, especially in advanced stages of the disease where they are usually associated with hemorrhages in the skin, lung, and gastrointestinal tract. Intracranial bleeding may occur in cerebral tissue, subarachnoid or subdural spaces, or in any combination of these sites. To a certain extent, the site of the hemorrhage is related to the factors causing the bleeding.

Thrombocytopenia

Thrombocytopenia is the main cause of bleeding in cancer patients. A marked increase in the tendency to bleed is seen for platelet counts lower than $20,000/mm^3$. Such low levels are fairly common after intensive chemotherapy or radiotherapy of large areas of bone marrow, following massive invasion of bone marrow by metastatic cells, and in patients with neoplasms originating from bone marrow cells, such as leukemias or multiple myeloma. Thrombocytopenia primarily causes subdural and subarachnoid hemorrhages, which may be partially prevented by platelet transfusions.

Cerebral Subdural Hematomas

Cerebral subdural hematomas are common in children with acute lymphocytic leukemia. They were found at autopsy in 13 of 126 leukemic children by Pitner and Johnson (1973). In this study, clinical symptoms consisted of increased intracranial pressure in nine cases, focal neurological signs (hemiparesis or paraparesis) in six, and seizures in five. Meningeal leukemia frequently coexisted with subdural hematomas. The authors suggest that chronic subdural hematoma should be suspected in children with acute lymphocytic leukemia and neurological symptoms who have no pleocytosis or blasts in the CSF and who do not respond to therapy for meningeal leukemia.

Spinal Subdural Hematomas

Spinal subdural hematomas are very rare compared to intracranial hematomas. They have been described in leukemic patients with thrombopenia after traumatic or difficult lumbar punctures (Wolcott et al., 1970; Edelson et al., 1974). Some spinal subdural hematomas have been discovered only at autopsy, whereas others have caused paraparesis, sensory loss, and/or urinary incontinence. These deficits may improve spontaneously and probably should not be treated by surgery or aspiration.

Vasculitis

In cancer patients, vasculitis, which increases vascular fragility, is mainly related to septicemia and hyperleukocytosis.

The incidence of septicemia increases markedly when the polymorphonuclear counts fall below 1,000 cells, particularly below 500 cells, per mm³. Infections in cancer patients are also favored by corticosteroid treatment and immunodepression, which is particularly marked in patients with lymphoma, leukemia, or myeloma. Hyperleukocytosis, which is capable of markedly increasing vascular fragility, is seen only in leukemia. In these patients, intracranial bleeding occurs in more than 50% of cases when leukocytosis exceeds 300,000 cells/mm³. Vascular lesions are due to the infiltration of vessel walls by blastic cells but more complex mechanisms may also be involved. Thus vasodilatation due to an increased nucleoprotein catabolism and hypoxia resulting from an increased blood viscosity eventually lead to bleeding in patients with hyperleukocytosis (Pochedly, 1975).

In leukemic patients, cerebral bleeding is usually multifocal. In cases with high leukocytosis, these foci are formed by leukemic cell nodules surrounded by hemorrhage.

Hemorrhages Caused by Metastases

The exact percentage of brain metastases producing massive hemorrhages is not known. A figure as high as 14% (13 of 92 cases) has been reported recently by Mandybur (1977). Intracranial bleeding occurs in large as well as in small brain metastases, most frequently in patients with melanoma, choriocarcinoma (Fig. 7.3), or lung carcinoma. In patients with small metastases, intracranial hemorrhage may be the first clinical manifestation of secondary brain tumors. Bleeding may involve any part of the brain. The onset of neurological signs is usually sudden but may be gradual. Hemorrhage may remain intracerebellar or break into the subarachnoid space, mimicking an aneurysm rupture, or into the ventricles. Bleeding of brain metastases, however, remains a rare cause of subarachnoid hemorrhage, observed in only 12 of 2,092 patients with subarachnoid hemorrhage reviewed by Locksley et al. (1966). Subdural hematomas may also develop as a result of bleeding of intracranial metastases (Russel and Cairns, 1934).

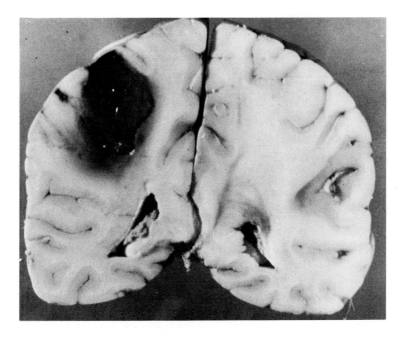

FIG. 7.3. Large hemorrhage within a metastasis of a choriocarcinoma. (Courtesy of Dr. J. Durant-Flament.)

The causes of bleeding of brain metastases are not clear. Rapidity of tumor growth, vascularization of the metastases, their tendency to invade vessels, embolizations, and necrosis have been considered as possible promoting factors. Where multiple metastases are present, hemorrhages may develop simultaneously in several tumors (Mandybur, 1977), suggesting that a hemorrhagic diathesis contributes to the bleeding of metastatic lesions. However, this explanation is speculative. In the majority of patients, the hemorrhages are spontaneous; in some cases, they are associated with radiotherapy or the administration of anticoagulant drugs, or provoked by head trauma. In cases with multiple metastases and intracranial bleeding, the prognosis is very poor. In patients with a single lesion located in accessible regions of the brain, however, surgical removal may improve the neurological status and prolong survival. In patients with chorioepithelioma, chemotherapy (methotrexate) should be used.

Intravascular Coagulation

Intravascular coagulation produces a variety of cerebrovascular lesions. A tendency toward bleeding results from thrombocytopenia, whereas cerebral embolisms may be due to NBTE, which occur in association with intravascular coagulation (Reagan and Okazaki, 1974). However, the most common cerebrovascular lesion of the intravascular coagulation is a thrombosis.

CEREBRAL THROMBOSIS, ISCHEMIA, AND HYPERVISCOSITY

Cerebral thrombosis, ischemia, and hyperviscosity may be related to the underlying neoplasm by the existence of a hypercoagulable state (intravascular coagulation), polycythemia, thrombocythemia, or serum hyperviscosity. Obstruction of vessels supplying the nervous system is also a major mechanism causing late neurological lesions due to irradiation. These complications are described in Chapter 5.

Intravascular Coagulation

Intravascular coagulation results from a hypercoagulable state, the cause of which is still poorly understood. Intravascular coagulation is associated with a variety of underlying diseases, including cancer, especially prostatic carcinoma, and acute myelocytic and promyelocytic leukemia. It is characterized by low levels of fibrinogen, the presence of fibrin degradation products, decreased prothrombin time, thrombopenia due to platelet consumption, and the presence of fragmented red cells in the peripheral blood. Multifocal cerebral infarcts may be caused by intravascular coagulation. The incidence of neurological manifestations in patients with intravascular coagulation is not known. In 45 patients with well-documented disseminated intravascular coagulation reported by Colman et al. (1972), the nervous system was not listed among the most frequently injured tissues. Twelve cases of intravascular coagulation with neurological lesions were found by Collins et al. (1975) in 1,459 autopsies. Ten patients had leukemia or lymphoma and two had breast carcinoma. Complete evaluation of the coagulation, however, was not available for all patients; in some, coagulation abnormalities were mild, and in five, neurological features preceded major changes of the coagulation tests.

Neurological Signs

Clinically, signs of generalized brain dysfunction consisting of confusion, disorientation, and delirium with agitation were found in all patients reported by Collins et al. (1975). In four cases, coma eventually developed. Four had generalized seizures, and two had asterixis or multifocal myoclonus. In addition focal signs of brain disease, such as focal seizures, hemiparesis, cortical blindness, aphasia, epilepsia partialis continua, or ataxia, were observed in seven patients.

Pathology

The pathology consists of multiple infarcts not exceeding 1 cm in diameter caused by fibrin thrombi. Such vessel obstructions are also found in other organs. Fresh multiple hemorrhages are frequently present, and subdural hematomas may be found. The differential diagnoses include metabolic encephalopathies in patients with diffuse brain dysfunctions and infarction and embolism or brain metastases in cases with focal brain signs.

Treatment

In the majority of patients with neurological lesions due to intravascular coagulation, the diagnosis was made at autopsy. It is therefore difficult to determine whether neurological deficits would respond to heparin administration, as do most of the extraneural lesions.

Polycythemia and Thrombocythemia

Polycythemia occurs as a primary disease (polycythemia vera or Osler-Vaquez disease) or in response to various stimuli listed in Table 7.2. Thrombocythemia is present in about 50% of patients with polycythemia vera. It is also found in other myeloproliferative disorders, such as myelofibrosis and chronic myelogenous leukemia, and rarely in association with certain neoplasms, such as lymphomas or bronchogenic carcinomas. Polycythemia and, to a much lesser extent, thrombocythemia contribute to create a state of hyperviscosity and hypervolemia which is responsible for a series of neurological disorders. Thrombocythemia plays a role in the pathogenesis of neurological abnormalities only when platelet aggregability is increased and when their count reaches $2.10^6/mm^3$.

Hyperviscosity and hypervolemia cause vascular distention, slowing of blood flow, stasis, and tissue hypoxia. Symptoms related to circulatory disturbances frequently involve the nervous system and have been best described in polycythemia vera.

Silverstein et al. (1962) reported neurological complications in 511 pa-

TABLE 7.2. *Causes of polycythemia*

A. Primary polycythemia (Osler-Vaquez disease)
B. Secondary polycythemia
    1. Generalized tissue hypoxia
    2. Renal lesions (local hypoxia)
        Hypernephroma, adenocarcinoma
        Cysts, polycystic kidneys
        Hydronephrosis
    3. Production of erythropoietine-like substance
        Cerebellar hemangioma
        Matrix fibroma
        Wilms tumor
        Pheochromocytoma
        Oat-cell lung carcinoma
        Cushing disease
        Hepatoma
    4. Excess of androgenic hormones

tients with polycythemia and reviewed the pertinent literature. Headache is the most frequent symptom, found in 35 to 85% of patients, dizziness or vertigo in 28 to 70%, visual disturbances, including scotoma, blurred vision, and papilledema, in 11 to 30%, paresthesia in about 15%, and tinnitus in less than 10%. All these symptoms are correlated with the values of the hematocrit and may regress partially or totally after adequate therapy.

Polycythemia and thrombocythemia also contribute to cerebrovascular strokes caused mainly by thrombosis and less frequently by cerebral hemorrhages, and to transient ischemic attacks. Considering the age of patients with polycythemia, one may argue that cerebrovascular complications seen in these patients are related to atherosclerosis. However, as pointed out by Gilbert (1975) for patients with polycythemia vera, cerebrosvascular accidents are four times more common than coronary artery disease, whereas the reverse is found in patients with atherosclerosis. Also, death is caused more frequently by cerebral than by coronary thrombosis in patients with polycythemia vera (Chievitz and Thiede, 1962). Adequate and rapid treatment of both primary and secondary polycythemia considerably reduces the incidence of vascular thromboembolic complications, including cerebrovascular disease.

Serum Hyperviscosity Syndrome

A marked rise of serum viscosity is seen in multiple myeloma, Waldenström disease, benign monoclonal gammopathy, and in diseases with immune system involvement, such as rheumatoid arthritis. Clinical manifestations of the serum hyperviscosity syndrome appear when the viscosity of the serum is higher than four times that of water (normal values range from 1.4 to 1.8) and for concentrations of the monoclonal globulin superior to 5 g/100 ml. However, there is no direct correlation between the serum viscosity and the appearance of clinical features. There are marked individual variations, probably related to predisposing factors, of the threshold at which clinical symptoms are seen. For instance, visual symptoms occur sooner in patients with predisposing diabetic retinopathy.

Clinical Features

Clinical manifestations are mainly of three types: general, vascular, and neurological. General symptoms consist of tiredness and loss of appetite. Vascular lesions cause epistaxis and hemorrhage of mucosae, mainly of the digestive tract. Neurological abnormalities include headache, nausea, dizziness, peripheral neuropathies, pain, and occasional seizures. Visual symptoms, such as scotoma, blurred vision, and loss of sight, are frequent manifestations of the serum hyperviscosity syndrome. Fund-eyes examinations may show thickened, sausage-shaped veins, flame-shaped hemorrhages, and papilledema.

Incidence of Serum Hyperviscosity Syndrome

The clinical hyperviscosity syndrome is commonly associated with Waldenström disease. In 25 patients with macroglobulinemia reviewed by Fahey et al. (1965), only seven were free of hyperviscosity manifestations. Neurological symptoms were found in 15 patients; five had vertigo and five others peripheral neuropathy. Ocular abnormalities were found in 11: all had retinal hemorrhage and three had loss of vision. The high incidence of clinical disorders caused by hyperviscosity in patients with Waldenström disease is attributed to physical properties of IgM found in this disease.

In IgG multiple myeloma, the hyperviscosity syndrome is found in about 4% of cases; it is more frequent in the IgG3 subclass (Hobbs, 1969; Pruzanski and Watt, 1972). In 10 patients with IgG myeloma and hyperviscosity syndrome described by Pruzanski and Watt (1972), all but two had fundus exudates and hemorrhages, and five had nervous system lesions. The hyperviscosity syndrome is considered to be rare in patients with IgA myeloma. However, the report of Tuddenham et al. (1974), although limited to four cases, suggests that the incidence of the hyperviscosity syndrome in IgA myeloma may be higher than previously suspected.

REFERENCES

Andersen, O. F., Fogelberg, M. G., Rosencrantz, N. M., Weinfeld, U. A., and Westin, J. E. (1977): Postlymphographic cerebral lipid embolization in the vena cava superior syndrome. *Cancer*, 39:79–84.

Barron, K. D., Siqueria, E., and Hirano, A. (1960): Cerebral embolism caused by nonbacterial thrombotic endocarditis. *Neurology,* 10:391–397.

Bryan, C. S. (1969): Nonbacterial thrombotic endocarditis with malignant tumors. *Am. J. Med.,* 46:787–793.

Burton, C., and Johnston, J. (1970): Multiple cerebral aneurysms and cardiac myxoma. *N. Engl. J. Med.,* 282:35–36.

Chievitz, E., and Thiede, T. (1962): Complications and causes of death in polycythaemia vera. *Acta Med. Scand.,* 172:513–523.

Chino, F., Kodama, A., Otake, M., and Dock, D. S. (1975): Nonbacterial thrombotic endocarditis in a Japanese autopsy sample. A review of eighty cases. *Am. Heart J.,* 90:190–196.

Collins, R. C., Al-Mondhiry, H., Chernik, N. L., and Posner, J. B. (1975): Neurologic manifestation of intravascular coagulation in patients with cancer. A clinicopathologic analysis of 12 cases. *Neurology,* 25:795–806.

Colman, R. W., Robboy, S. J., and Minna, J. D. (1972): Desseminated intravascular coagulation (DIC): An approach. *Am. J. Med.,* 52:679–689.

Damasio, H., Seabra-Gomes, R., Da Silva, J. P., Damasio, A. R., and Antunes, J. L. (1975): Multiple cerebral aneurysms and cardiac myxoma. *Arch. Neurol.,* 32:269–270.

Edelson, R. N., Chernik, N. L., and Posner, J. B. (1974): Spinal subdural hematomas complicating lumbar puncture. *Arch. Neurol.,* 31:134–137.

Fahey, J. L., Barth, W. F., and Salomon, A. (1965): Serum hyperviscosity syndrome. *JAMA,* 192:464–467.

Gilbert, H. S. (1975): Definition, clinical features and diagnosis of polycythaemia vera. *Clin. Haematol.,* 4:263–290.

Greenwood, W. F. (1968): Profile of atrial myxoma. *Am. J. Cardiol.,* 21:367–375.

Hobbs, J. R. (1969): Immunochemical clones of myelomatosis. *Br. J. Haematol.,* 16: 599–606.

Locksley, B. H., Sahs, A. L., and Sander, R. (1966): Report on the cooperative study of intracranial aneurysms and arachnoid hemorrhage. Section III. Subarachnoid hemorrhage unrelated to intracranial aneurysm and A-V malformations. *J. Neurosurg.,* 26:1034–1056.

MacDonald, R. A., and Robbins, S. L. (1957): The significance of nonbacterial thrombotic endocarditis: An autopsy and clinical study of 78 cases. *Ann. Intern. Med.,* 46: 255–273.

Mandybur, T. I. (1977): Intracranial hemorrhage caused by metastatic tumors. *Neurology,* 27:650–655.

Pitner, S. E., and Johnson, W. W. (1973): Chronic subdural hematoma in childhood acute leukemia. *Cancer,* 32:185–190.

Pochedly, C. (1975): Neurologic manifestations in acute leukemia. I. Symptoms due to increased cerebrospinal final pressure and hemorrhage. *NY State J. Med.,* 75: 575–580.

Price, D. L., Harris, J. L., New, P. F. J., and Cantu, R. C. (1970): Cardiac myxoma. A clinicopathologic and angiographic study. *Arch. Neurol.,* 23:558–567.

Pruzanski, W., and Watt, J. G. (1972): Serum viscosity and hyperviscosity syndrome in IgG multiple myeloma. Report of 10 patients and review of the literature. *Ann. Int. Med.,* 77:853–860.

Reagan, T. J., and Okazaki, H. (1974): The thrombotic syndrome associated with carcinoma. *Arch. Neurol.,* 31:390–395.

Rosen, P., and Armstrong, D. (1973): Nonbacterial thrombotic endocarditis in patients with malignant neoplastic diseases. *Am. J. Med.,* 54:23–29.

Russel, D. S., and Cairns, H. (1934): Subdural false membrane of hematoma (pachymeningitis interna haemorrhagica) in carcinomatosis and sarcomatosis of the dura mater. *Brain,* 57:32–48.

Schwartz, G. A., Schwartzman, R. J., and Joyner, C. (1972): Atrial myxoma. Cause of embolic stroke. *Neurology,* 22:1112–1121.

Silverstein, A., Gilbert, H., and Wasserman, L. R. (1962): Neurologic complications of polycythaemia. *Ann. Intern. Med.,* 57:909–916.

Stoane, L., Allen, J. H., Jr., and Collins, H. A. (1966): Radiologic observations in cerebral embolism. *Radiology,* 87:262–266.

Tuddenham, E. G. D., Whittaker, J. A., Bradley, J., Lilleman, J. S., and James, D. R. (1974): Hyperviscosity syndrome in IgA. Multiple myeloma. *Br. J. Haematol.,* 27: 65–76.

Weinstein, L., and Schlesinger, J. J. (1974): Pathoanatomic, pathophysiologic and clinical correlation in endocarditis (second of two parts). *N. Engl. J. Med.,* 291:1122–1126.

Wolcott, G. J., Grunnet, M. L., and Lahey, E. (1970): Spinal subdural hematoma in a leukemic child. *J. Pediatr.,* 77:1060–1062.

Wolman, L., and Bradshaw, P. (1967): Spinal cord embolism. *J. Neurol. Neurosurg. Psychiatry,* 30:446–454.

Yufe, R., Karpati, G., and Carpenter, S. (1976): Cardiac myxoma: A diagnostic challenge for the neurologist. *Neurology (Minneap.),* 26:1060–1065.

Chapter 8

Carcinomatous Neuropathies

The so-called carcinomatous neuropathies form a group of rare neurological diseases attributed to a remote effect of cancer on the nervous system. A guide for their classification, based on clinicopathological data, was established in 1965 by the late Lord Brain and R. Adams. This guide is still valid today (Table 8.1) because little progress has been made since then in understanding the pathogenesis of these diseases. In particular, their relationship to cancer remains unexplained. One of these, however, progressive multifocal leukoencephalopathy, was attributed to papovavirus and is presently considered one of the infectious complications of neoplastic diseases.

If one considers the remote effects of cancer, one can distinguish two general classes. The first, represented by, e.g., weight loss, anemia, or infections, can be explained by factors not specific for cancer. The second group, the so-called paraneoplasias, is quite different. They are specifically caused by an

TABLE 8.1. *Classification of carcinomatous neuropathies*

Syndrome	Relative frequency	Location of main lesions	Main associated neoplasms
Metabolic encephalopathies	Fairly frequent		Oat-cell lung carcinoma when caused by production of active substances by the tumor
Diffuse polyencephalo-myelitis	Rare	Limbic system; brainstem; spinal cord	Oat-cell lung carcinoma
Subacute cerebellar degeneration	Rare	Degeneration of Purkinje cells	Oat-cell lung carcinoma; ovary carcinoma
Opsoclonus	Rare	Cerebellum (?); brainstem (?)	Neuroblastoma
Motor neuron disease	Very rare	Degeneration of spinal motor neurons	Lung and breast carcinomas
Necrotizing myelopathy	Very rare	Spinal (mainly thoracic) cord	Lung carcinoma
Sensory neuropathy	Rare	Root, ganglia, and spinal cord	Lung carcinoma
Sensorimotor peripheral neuropathy	Frequent	Peripheral nerves	Lung and breast carcinomas
Eaton-Lambert syndrome	Fairly rare	Neuromuscular junction	Oat-cell lung carcinoma
Muscle lesions			
Neuromyopathy	The most frequent	Proximal muscles and peripheral nerves (?)	Mainly lung and breast carcinomas
Polymyositis and dermatomyositis	Fairly rare	Muscles	Lung, breast, ovary, lymphomas
Carcinoid syndrome myopathy	Very rare	Muscles	Serotonin-secreting tumors

abnormal function of cancer tissue, such as the production of hormones or hormone-like proteins. To which of these classes do the carcinomatous neuropathies belong? An example of a remote effect of cancer on nervous tissue is the production of the nerve-growth factor by mice (Levi-Montalcini, 1952) and also human sarcoma (Waddell et al., 1972). But none of the described cancerous neuropathies can be explained by this mechanism.

Many if not all syndromes forming the group of carcinomatous neuropathies are also observed in patients without cancer. There is no correlation between the response to treatment of the neuropathy and that of the underlying malignancy and no correlation between the extent of the neoplasm and the severity of neurological disorders. Frequently, the neuropathy was diagnosed years before the discovery of the malignant disease. The relationship between the so-called carcinomatous neuropathies and cancer is thus based on the alleged frequency of their association, which is considered separately for each syndrome.

METABOLIC ENCEPHALOPATHIES

Disorientation, mental changes, confusion, and alterations of consciousness seen in patients with cancer are frequently related to metabolic disorders. These are essentially of two types.

The first group represents truly paraneoplastic syndromes. They are due to derepression, which occurs in certain neoplastic cells. This derepression results in the production by the tumors, mainly the oat-cell carcinoma, of hormones or hormone-like substances (Table 8.2). The main characteristic

TABLE 8.2. *Main causes of metabolic encephalopathies in patients with cancer*

Metabolic abnormalities	Paraneoplasic syndromes, tumor secretion of	Other causes related to cancer
Hypercalcemia	Parathormone; parathormone-like substance; prostaglandins E	Bone metastases; multiple myeloma
Hypokalemia	ACTH	Malabsorption due to carcinomatous or postradiation lesions of mesenteric lymphatics
Hypernatremia	ACTH	Hemoconcentration
Hyponatremia	Antidiuretic hormone (Schwartz-Barter syndrome)	Vincristine and cyclophosphamide treatment
Hypoglycemia	Insulin; insulin-like hormone	Glucose consumption by the tumor (?)
Uremia	—	Nephrotoxic chemotherapy (methotrexate); obstruction of urinary tract by tumor
Anoxia	—	Pulmonary primary and metastatic tumors; pulmonary infection; anemia
Hepatic failure	—	Liver primary and metastatic tumors; hepatoxic chemotherapy (*l*-asparaginase)

of these paraneoplastic manifestations is their reversibility when the tumor is adequately treated.

The second group of metabolic encephalopathies seen in cancer patients is due to a variety of mechanisms (Table 8.2), including the invasion of vital organs (e.g., liver, mesenteric lymphatics, urinary tract, lung, and bones), liver or kidney dysfunction due to certain chemotherapeutic drugs, or inappropriate secretion of the antidiuretic hormone due to the administration of some chemotherapeutic agents.

DIFFUSE POLIOENCEPHALOMYELITIS

Histological examination of the nervous system in patients with diffuse polioencephalomyelitis strongly suggests that multiple clinical manifestations are actually part of the same pathological entity. The most common clinical presentations of this disease are limbic encephalitis, brainstem encephalitis, and myelitis. The most prominent neurological features of carcinomatous polioencephalomyelitis are related to the localization of the most severe histological lesions. However, the pathological abnormalities are usually widespread and extend far beyond the area that determines the most conspicuous clinical signs. Therefore, transitory forms are frequent. Two additional carcinomatous neuropathies are often associated with diffuse polioencephalomyelitis: the subacute cerebellar degeneration and the sensory neuropathy first described by Denny-Brown (1948); they are considered separately.

Clinical Signs and Complementary Examinations

Clinical manifestations of 30 cases of carcinomatous polioencephalomyelitis reported in the world literature have been reviewed by Dorfman and Forno (1972). The disease occurs most commonly between the ages of 50 and 70 years and has no definite sex predominance. The duration of the illness ranges from 2 to 24 months, with an average length of 10 months. Patients are afebrile. The most common and most striking neurological feature is a rapidly progressive dementia with early memory disturbances. Mental changes, consisting of anxiety, agitation, hallucinations, or depression, have been reported in 23 of 28 cases of encephalitis associated with carcinoma reviewed by Kaplan and Itabashi (1974).

In patients with brainstem involvement, external ophthalmoplegia, nystagmus, and gaze paralysis are seen when the lesions predominate in the upper brainstem, whereas bulbar palsies are frequent in lower brainstem injuries. Ataxia seen in these patients should be attributed to cerebellar degeneration, which is frequently associated with brainstem polioencephalitis. Myelitis is characterized by weakness and muscle atrophy since lesions primarily involved the motor neurons. Symptoms of myelitis may be seen alone, without signs of lesions at upper levels. The lesions may be restricted to a segment of the spinal cord producing, for instance, a cervical and bibrachial palsy (case records of Massachusetts General Hospital, 1970).

Cerebrospinal fluid (CSF) may be normal, but protein and cell counts are usually elevated. In Dorfman and Forno's review (1972), protein levels higher than 60 mg/100 ml (average 160 mg/100 ml) were found in 17 of 26 cases, and increased cell counts (mean value 34 cells/mm^3) in 17 of 24 cases. The EEG shows diffuse, noncharacteristic abnormalities. Radiographic contrast studies are normal.

Pathology

Microscopic lesions of the central nervous systems (CNS) are widespread but frequently predominate in the limbic system (hippocampal formation and amygdaloid nuclei), orbital cortex, brainstem, and ventral horns of the medullary cord. Microscopically, the lesions consist of an inflammatory reaction: lymphocytic infiltrates of the meninges, parenchymal glial nodules, and perivascular (mainly perivenous) lymphocytic cupping (Figs. 8.1 and 8.2). The inflammatory reaction often appears disproportionate to the degenerative neuronal changes. Electron microscopic examinations, which were performed in a few cases, failed to demonstrate the presence of viral particles.

Relationship with Cancer and Pathogenesis

This type of polioencephalomyelitis is not seen exclusively in patients with cancer. Limbic encephalitis closely resembling the carcinomatous polioencephalitis was originally described as a separate entity. The fact that the association between polioencephalitis and cancer has been emphasized in the literature during the last 20 years may simply reflect the interest raised by carcinomatous neuropathies. Diffuse polioencephalomyelitis is rare, even in patients with malignant tumors, where it is associated primarily with bronchogenic oat-cell carcinoma and especially with tumors of ovary, uterus, or stomach. Pathological features strongly suggest a viral etiology, but the evidence of this pathogenesis has not yet been established.

SUBACUTE CEREBELLAR DEGENERATION

The subacute cerebellar degeneration frequently associated with diffuse polioencephalomyelitis is often described as part of this entity. However, the main pathological characteristic of diffuse polioencephalomyelitis is a widespread inflammatory reaction, which is not seen in carcinomatous cerebellar degeneration. For this reason, the syndrome is described separately.

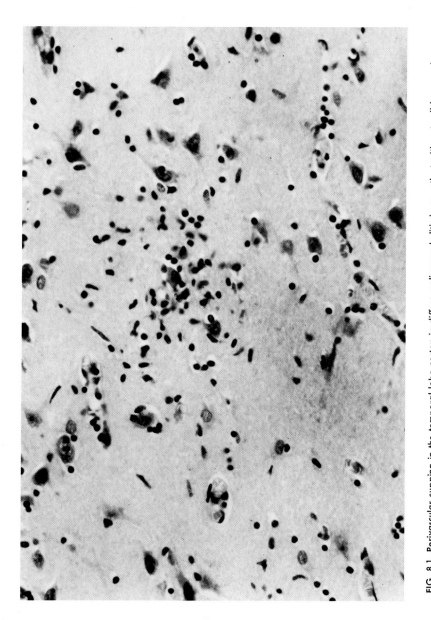

FIG. 8.1. Perivascular cupping in the temporal lobe cortex in diffuse polioencephalitis in a patient with oat-cell lung carcinoma. (Courtesy of Dr. J. J. Vanderhaeghen.)

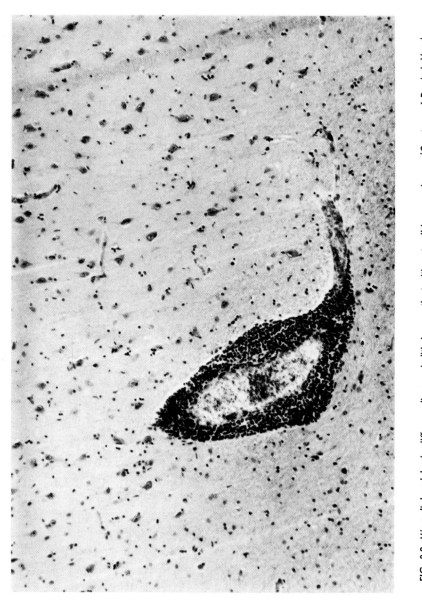

FIG. 8.2. Microglial nodules in diffuse polioencephalitis in a patient with oat-cell lung carcinoma. (Courtesy of Dr. J. J. Vander-haeghen.)

Clinical Signs and CSF Changes

Subacute cerebellar degeneration is often associated with a diffuse polio-encephalomyelitis and/or sensory neuropathy. Therefore, mental changes, motor signs, such as ptosis and facial or limb weakness, sensory symptoms, loss or diminished tendon reflexes, and Babinski signs, are found quite often in these patients (Brain and Wilkinson, 1965a). Cerebellar signs include ataxia, present in all patients reviewed by Brain and Wilkinson (1965b). In all but two cases, there was ataxia in both the upper and lower limbs. Dysarthria was present in 15 of 19 patients. Nystagmus was marked in five patients, slight in four, and absent in 10 others. CSF may be normal; but of 13 cases, protein was increased in five, ranging from 60 to 120 mg/100 ml; cell number was increased in two patients.

Pathology

Pathologically, the disease is characterized by the disappearance of the Purkinje cells in the cerebellar cortex (Fig. 8.3). In contrast to the cerebellar cortical degeneration occurring in alcoholic patients (Victor et al., 1959), the cerebellar degeneration seen in cancer patients is diffuse. There is no inflammatory reaction in the cerebellar cortex, but inflammation may be seen in deep structures of the cerebellum (Fig. 8.4). Some degenerative changes may be seen in the molecular and granular layers.

Relationship with Cancer and Pathogenesis

Subacute cerebellar degeneration, clinically and pathologically similar to that associated with cancer, may be seen in patients without malignant diseases (Monseu et al., 1971). As the association of several other forms of neuropathies with malignancy, that of cerebellar degeneration may be biased to some extent by the interest generated by these diseases. Of 19 cases reviewed by Brain and Wilkinson (1965a), neurological disorders preceded the discovery of neoplasm in 12 patients. The interval ranged from 2 to 96 months, and the assumption that malignant disease was actually present 2 to 3 years or even more before its discovery remains speculative. Subacute cerebellar degeneration seen in cancer patients is mainly associated with carcinoma of lung and ovary (Monseu et al., 1971). The mechanism of the remote effect of cancer on the cerebellum, if it exists, remains unexplained.

OPSOCLONUS

Clinical Signs

Opsoclonus consists of abnormal, continuous lightning eye movements generally taking place on a horizontal plane. The chaotic and irregular char-

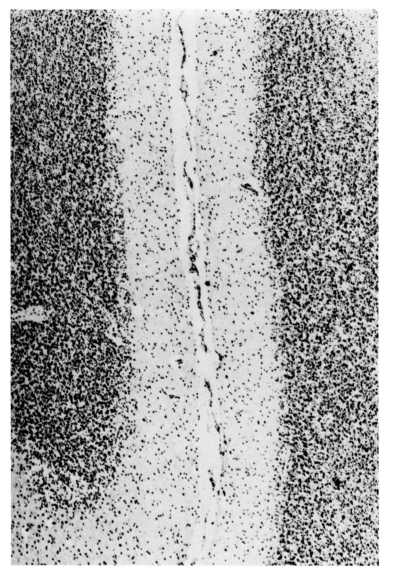

FIG. 8.3. Complete disappearance of Purkinje cells in the cerebellar hemisphere in a case of subacute cerebellar degeneration associated with lung carcinoma. (Courtesy of Dr. J. J. Vanderhaegen.)

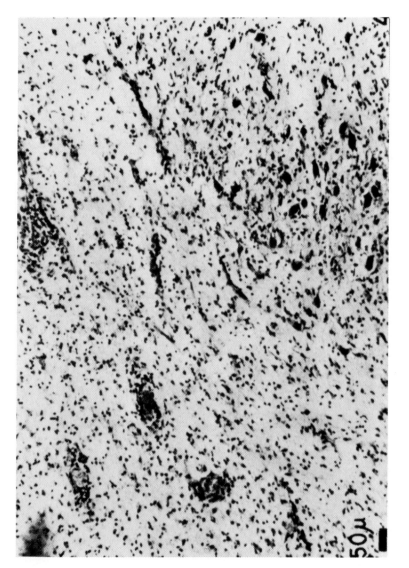

FIG. 8.4. Inflammatory reaction in deep cerebellar structures in a case of subacute degeneration associated with lung carcinoma. (Courtesy of Dr. J. J. Vanderhaegen.)

acter of eye movements contrasts with the rhythmicity of nystagmus. The pathological basis of opsoclonus remains unclear. Opsoclonus has been observed in patients with cerebellar diseases (Ellenberger et al., 1968), encephalitis characterized by lymphocytic infiltration predominating in the hypothalamus, midbrain, and pons, and also in a patient with unexitable labyrinths due to streptomycin toxicity (Cogan, 1954).

Relationship with Cancer and Pathogenesis

The possibility of a relationship between opsoclonus and neoplasms was first considered by Allesi in 1940. In 1967, Ross and Zeman described a patient with lung carcinoma who had opsoclonus, cerebellar degeneration, and diffuse but mild polioencephalitis characterized by perivascular lymphocytic infiltrations. However, the most intriguing association is that of opsoclonus with occult neuroblastoma (Solomon and Chutorian, 1968; Senelick et al., 1973). In some cases, however, neuroblastoma may be heralded by cerebellar signs without opsoclonus (Moe and Nellhaus, 1970; Roberts and Freeman, 1975). In the case reported by Moe and Nellhaus (1970), opsoclonus appeared only after operation for neuroblastoma. The nature of the relationship between opsoclonus and neuroblastoma is not understood.

AMYOTROPHIC LATERAL SCLEROSIS

Clinical Signs and Pathology

The clinical features of amyotrophic lateral sclerosis (ALS) result from a combination of signs caused by lower motor neuron lesions with those caused by the degeneration of corticobulbar and corticospinal tracts. One finds, therefore, progressive bulbar palsy and/or predominantly distal limb weakness and muscle atrophy, fasciculations, and fibrillations due to the lower motor neuron disease. Pseudobulbar palsy, spasticity, increase in tendon reflexes and Babinski signs are caused by the upper motor neuron lesions. Mental and sensory changes are absent; CSF is normal.

ALS syndrome reported in patients with cancer is essentially similar to the classic ALS, with some differences. In patients with cancer, the male predominance was greater and their mean age more than a decade higher than in patients without neoplasm (Norris and Engel, 1965). In the study of Brain et al. (1965), the motor neuron disease appeared more benign and self-limiting in patients with cancer. The pathological findings are typical of classical ALS.

Relationship with Cancer and Pathogenesis

In the study of Norris and Engel (1965), ALS associated with cancer represents 10% of 130 consecutive cases of lower motor neuron lesions seen by these authors. This percentage is exceptionally high and has not been confirmed by other authors. In 186 patients with ALS reported by Shy and Silverstein (1965), nine (4.8%) had cancer, whereas none of 80 autopsied patients with ALS reported by Rowland (1965) had a malignant tumor. Of 11 patients with cancer and ALS reported by Brain et al. (1965), three cases were found during a routine examination of almost 1,500 cancer patients, indicating that the disease is rarely associated with malignancy. Of 24 cases reported in the studies of Brain et al. (1965) and Norris and Engel (1965), the most common tumor sites were lung (eight cases) and breast (four cases). As for many other rare forms of the so-called carcinomatous neuropathies, pathogenesis of carcinomatous ALS remains unexplained.

NECROTIZING MYELOPATHY

Necrotizing myelopathy, a very rare disease, is characterized by an acute or subacute paraplegia, which is usually somewhat spastic at its onset and becomes rapidly flaccid and areflectic. The lesions predominate at the thoracic level. Sensory loss is present below the lesion. Paralysis of bladder and rectum are common. The neurological deficit is irreversible. CSF protein levels were increased in five of six cases where levels were determined.

Pathology

With the exception of two cases, histological lesions are restricted to the spinal cord, which may be swollen in a fusiform fashion. Massive or patchy necrosis affects both gray and white matter. It often predominates in central and dorsal areas and extends through many segments. There is no inflammatory or glial reaction.

Relationship with Cancer and Pathogenesis

Seven cases were collected by Mancall and Rosales in 1964; most were associated with lung carcinoma. Since then, two cases of necrotizing myelopathy were observed in association with lymphomas (Richter and Moore, 1968) and one with ovary carcinoma (case records of Massachusetts General Hospital, 1976). The relationship between necrotic myelopathy and cancer remains unclarified.

SENSORY NEUROPATHY

Clinical Signs

Sensory neuropathy applies to a disorder in which sensory abnormalities are dominant. Paresthesia, which may be very distressing, loss of all forms of sensibility, and ataxia of sensory origin are the major symptoms. They develop progressively during a period of a few months and then usually remain stationary. Sensory deficits predominate in the lower limbs. They may be asymmetrical. Pseudoathetosis, consisting of irregular, involuntary movements of fingers, is common (Croft et al., 1965).

In addition to symptoms caused by sensory lesions, other neurological signs, such as mental abnormalities, muscle weakness and atrophy, extensor plantar responses, and bladder disturbances, have been observed. CSF protein is frequently raised.

Pathology

The main lesions are found in root ganglia where destruction of a large number of cells is present together with a scattered inflammatory reaction. In the spinal cord, there is a Wallerian degeneration and demyelination of posterior columns secondary to ganglia lesions. In addition, inflammatory reactions similar to that which characterizes diffuse polioencephalomyelitis may be found in the spinal cord, brainstem, and limbic system, suggesting an intimate connection between sensory neuropathy and other forms of carcinomatous polioencephalomyelitis (Croft et al., 1965).

Relationship with Cancer and Pathogenesis

The two first cases of sensory neuropathy associated with bronchogenic carcinomas were described by Denny-Brown in 1948. Since then, the association of this neuropathy with lung cancer—particularly oat-cell carcinoma—has been confirmed. The pathogenesis of the disease and its relationship with the underlying malignancy remain unexplained. The presence of serum antibodies reacting with human brain tissue was investigated in patients with various types of carcinomatous neuropathies by Wilkinson (1964) using the complement-fixation test and by Wilkinson and Zeromski (1965) using immunofluorescent techniques. Only patients with sensory neuropathies showed positive results. These findings do not necessarily indicate that sensory neuropathy is a primary immunological disease; pathologically, it differs from autoimmune neurological diseases, such as allergic encephalomyelitis or allergic polyneuritis. In addition, the presence of antibodies may be the result rather than the cause of nervous tissue damage. Nevertheless, sensory neuropathy is the only carcinomatous neuropathy where such antibodies were found with high frequency.

PERIPHERAL SENSORIMOTOR NEUROPATHY

Clinical Signs

Sensorimotor polyneuritis occurring in cancer patients is similar to peripheral neuropathies of other etiologies. The symptoms usually predominate in the lower limbs and consist of symmetrical paresthesia, depression of myotatic reflexes, distal muscle weakness and atrophy, and sensory changes. In myeloma, painful neuropathies are present in approximately 60% of patients and may be very debilitating (Davis and Drachman, 1972). Few cases of Guillain-Barré syndrome have been observed in association with cancer (Klingon, 1965; Powles and Malpas, 1967).

Pathology

Examinations of sural nerve biopsies obtained from patients with confirmed malignant tumors (Schlaepfer, 1974) revealed acute axonal degeneration and a relative increase of small myelinated fibers. Sequential demyelination is very rare. The magnitude of these lesions is roughly correlated with the degree of clinical polyneuritis.

Relationship with Cancer and Pathogenesis

In studies where the incidence of carcinomatous neuropathies was evaluated in unselected patients with cancer, sensorimotor polyneuropathy accounted for 19% of all forms of carcinomatous neuropathies (Croft and Wilkinson, 1965). They are particularly frequent in patients with lung cancer, where they were observed in 20% of cases (Croft and Wilkinson, 1965).

The causes of peripheral neuropathy are numerous. One must determine whether the lesions of peripheral nerves found in patients with cancer are due to a remote effect of the neoplasia or result from nonspecific causes, such as vitamins or alimentary deficiences, or treatments by neurotoxic drugs, which are more frequent in cancer patients than in a general population.

In a prospective study where neuromuscular biopsies and EMG were performed in 50 consecutive cancer patients, we (Hildebrand and Coers, 1967) found that in the absence of clinical evidence of nutritional deficiency, there was no indication of clinical or even subclinical neuromuscular disorders. In association with malnutrition, however, a high proportion of histological abnormalities was found.

The opinion that polyneuropathies seen in patients with cancer are not related to malignancy by a specific mechanism is further supported by the study of Wilner and Brody (1968). They found that unexplained neurological signs were at least as high among patients with chronic nonneoplastic pulmonary diseases as in patients with lung cancer.

Peripheral Neuropathies in Myeloma

The peripheral neuropathies seen in patients with myeloma are of two types: one with and one without amyloidosis. The latter variety, which represents a form of carcinomatous polyneuritis, is of particular interest. It is seen primarily in osteosclerotic myeloma, which represents only about 3% of all cases of myeloma (Davis and Drachman, 1972; Mangalik and Veliath, 1971; case records of Massachusetts General Hospital, 1972, 1977). Symmetrical polyneuropathy occurs in about 30 to 35% of patients with osteosclerotic myeloma. A syndrome combining severe polyneuropathy, osteosclerotic myeloma, gynecomastia, and hirsutism was first noted by Waldenström (1976) and recently confirmed in a number of Japanese patients. The high percentage of patients with osteosclerotic myeloma in whom peripheral neuropathy is found and the improvement of the neurological signs develop after radiotherapy (Davis and Drachman, 1972) strongly suggests a remote effect of the neoplasia on the nervous system in this particular malignancy.

EATON-LAMBERT SYNDROME

Clinical and Electrophysiological Features

The Eaton-Lambert syndrome, sometimes referred to as the myasthenic syndrome, is essentially different from myasthenia gravis (Table 8.3). It is usually seen in males over 40 years of age. It consists of proximal weakness and fatigue, which predominate in the lower limbs, producing gait abnormalities and difficulties in getting up from a sitting position or climbing stairs. Strength may be increased by repetition of movements. Muscle wasting is not prominent. Myotatic reflexes are frequently depressed and may be abolished. Ptosis, diplopia, and dysphagia are rare and are mild when present. CSF is normal. Muscle response to nerve stimulation is characteristic: the response to a single stimulus is reduced, and a marked facilitation is seen after repetitive stimulations at 10 to 50 cycles/sec (Fig. 8.5).

The defect of neuromuscular transmission in Eaton-Lambert syndrome

TABLE 8.3. *Comparison between Eaton-Lambert syndrome and myasthenia gravis*

Factor	Eaton-Lambert syndrome	Myasthenia gravis
Age and sex	Males over 40 years	Young females
Associated tumors	Malignant tumors in 70% (oat-cell lung carcinoma)	Thymoma in 50%
Main location of weakness	Proximal segments of limbs	Oculobulbar muscles
Electromyography (repetitive nerve stimulation, 10 to 50 cycles/sec)	Facilitation: increase of evoked muscle potentials	Fatigue: decrease of evoked muscle potentials
Anomaly of the neuromuscular junction	Impaired release of acetylcholine	Antibodies against acetylcholine receptors
Drug effect		
Anticholinesterases	Ineffective	Effective
Decamethonium (1.5 to 2.5 mg)	Produces a more marked weakness in patients with Eaton-Lambert syndrome than in controls	Produces a less marked weakness in patients with myasthenia gravis than in controls
Guanidine	Effective	Poor

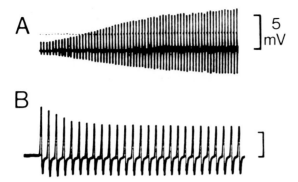

FIG. 8.5. A: Facilitation (increment) of the successive evoked muscle potentials recorded in abductor pollicis in a patient with Eaton-Lambert syndrome. The stimulation of the median nerve was applied at the wrist at 20 cycles/sec. The amplitude of the initial potential is markedly reduced. B: Decrement of the successive evoked muscle potentials recorded in the abductor pollicis in a patient with myasthenia gravis. The stimulation of the cubital nerve was applied at the wrist at 20 cycles/sec. The amplitude of the initial potential is normal. The speed of the recording film is different in the two examinations. (Courtesy of Dr. S. Borenstein.)

consists of a reduction in the acetylcholine vesicles released at the motor nerve endings. Magnesium, neomycin, and botulism toxin, which decrease the release of acetylcholine, produce symptoms similar to those of Eaton-Lambert syndrome. The syndrome is improved by guanidine, which increases the release of acetylcholine, whereas anticholinesterases are ineffective.

Pathology

Muscle biopsies performed in 20 patients with Eaton-Lambert syndrome (Lambert and Rooke, 1965) were normal in 11 cases. Nine had nonspecific alterations consisting of degenerative changes in variable numbers of muscle fibers, scattered atrophic fibers, and perivascular round cells found in two cases. Changes of the axonal membrane in the neuromuscular junction have been demonstrated by electron microscopy (Fukumara et al., 1972).

Relationship with Cancer and Pathogenesis

Eaton-Lambert syndrome satisfies several criteria of a truly paraneoplastic disease resulting from a remote effect of cancer on the neuromuscular junction. The syndrome is not rare in an unselected population of cancer patients, where it accounts for 9% of all carcinomatous neuropathies (Croft and Wilkinson, 1965). Conversely, in patients with Eaton-Lambert syndrome, malignant tumors are frequently found. For instance, of 40 patients with this syndrome seen at the Mayo Clinic, 28 (70%) had malignant tumors, of which 20 were small cell lung carcinomas.

Another interesting feature of this syndrome is its ability to respond, at least in some cases, to treatment of the neoplasm (Norris et al., 1965).

Finally, an acetone extract of cancer tissue from a patient with Eaton-Lambert syndrome has been shown (Ishikawa et al., 1977) to reduce the acetylcholine release from motor nerve endings and to produce a defect in neuromuscular transmission in the frog nerve-muscle preparation.

MUSCULAR LESIONS

Primary muscular lesions observed in cancer patients have been described as neuromyopathy or neuromuscular syndrome, polymyositis, and myopathy. Clinically, the syndromes to which these designations refer are different. Pathologically, however, they are all characterized by the necrosis of muscle fibers, the importance of which varies considerably from one case to another, and a comparatively discreet inflammatory reaction. The pathogenesis of muscular lesions of patients bearing malignant tumors has not been elucidated. Therefore, it has not yet been established whether or not the muscular diseases described under various designations in patients with neoplastic disease are part of the same entity.

NEUROMYOPATHY OR NEUROMUSCULAR SYNDROME

Clinical Signs

The term neuromyopathy designates a syndrome defined by Shy and Silverstein (1965) that combines signs of neuropathy, such as decrease of myotatic reflexes, with progressive, symmetrical, proximal weakness of body-supporting muscles. The main complaint of these patients is difficulty standing, rising from a sitting position, and climbing stairs. Electromyographic studies often show myopathic lesions. Short polyphasic potentials are markedly increased in some patients.

Pathology

Muscle biopsies demonstrate changes suggestive of myopathic lesions (Shy and Silverstein, 1965): loss of cross striations; flocular, cloudy, granular changes; internally placed nuclei; and increase of endomysial connective tissue. In addition, basophilic fibers containing large nuclei and prominent nucleoli characteristic of regeneration of muscles were seen in some cases. Inflammatory cell infiltrations are rare and scanty in neuromyopathy of patients with cancer.

Relationship with Cancer

The incidence of neuromyopathy, or neuromuscular syndrome, which accounts for 65% of all carcinomatous neuropathies in an unselected population of cancer patients (Croft and Wilkinson, 1965) was assessed by Shy and

Silverstein (1965). In a series of 1,500 patients hospitalized for a variety of malignancies at the National Cancer Institute, the incidence of this syndrome was only 3.5%. Conversely, in patients presenting with a proximal symmetrical weakness who came to a neurologist, 18.5% had malignant tumors. In patients over 50 years of age, this incidence climbs to 33.4% and to 60% when only males are taken into account. It is thus in males over 50 years old that the remote effect of cancer on the neuromuscular apparatus is best indicated by statistical data.

POLYMYOSITIS AND DERMATOMYOSITIS

Polymyositis is an inflammatory disease of muscle tissue. In dermatomyositis, there is in addition inflammation of the skin, producing a characteristic rash. The cause of these disorders is unknown. The clinical features of polymyositis and dermatomyositis associated with malignancy do not differ from those occurring in patients without cancer.

Clinical Signs, Electromyography, and Laboratory Data

Polymyositis and dermatomyositis are characterized by proximal muscular weakness progressing over weeks or months, with spontaneous remissions and exacerbations. The strength of facial and distal limb muscles may be slightly diminished or remain normal. Tendon reflexes remain evocable. Muscular pain, tenderness, and swelling are common. Dysphagia is frequent, and weakness of respiratory muscles may occur. Raynaud phenomenon is found in about 30%.

In dermatomyositis, the rash is characterized by lilac discoloration of upper eyelids, periorbital edema, erythema, dermal atrophy, and red patches. The typical distribution of skin lesions involves the knuckles, elbows, knees, medial malleoli, face, neck, and upper chest and back.

Electromyography is characterized by (a) spontaneous fibrillation potentials, which tend to disappear when the disease improves, and (b) polyphasic but short and small motor unit potentials and high frequency repetitive discharges. Sarcoplasmic enzymes, creatine phosphokinase, aldolase, transaminases, and lactic dehydrogenase are increased in the serum of most patients with polymyositis. However, the enzymatic activities may remain normal even in patients with active polymyositis (Bohan and Peter, 1975). Serum gamma globulins are raised in about 20% of cases. Sedimentation rate is increased more frequently in patients with cancer than in an unselected population of patients with polymyositis.

Pathology

The pathological changes include focal or diffuse necrosis of muscle fibers, regenerative activity reflected by basophilia of same fibers, and an inflamma-

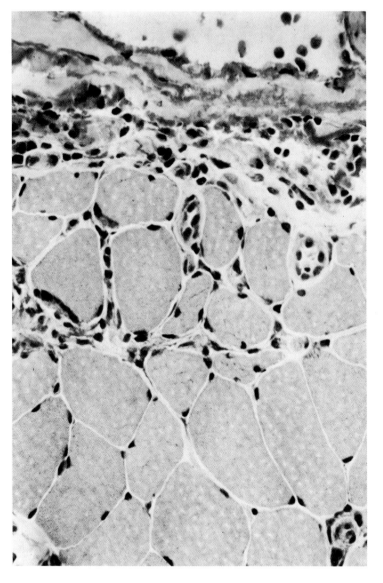

FIG. 8.6. Perivascicular atrophy and interstitial inflammatory reaction (lymphocyte infiltration) in a patient with a polymyositis associated with ovary carcinoma. The degenerative changes are scanty. (Courtesy of Dr. C. Coers.)

tory reaction characterized by the infiltration of fibers of perivascular spaces with lymphocytes and plasma cells. When myositis is present in cancer patients, the lymphocytic reaction is generally poor, but there are frequent exceptions (Fig. 8.6). In some cases, the disproportion between the extent of muscle fiber necrosis and the lack of inflammatory lymphocytic exudate is such that diagnosis is that of muscle necrosis (Smith, 1968; Swash, 1974). Whether such cases represent a variety of myositis or a form of myopathy remains an open question (Urich and Wilkinson, 1970).

Relationship with Cancer and Pathogenesis

Polymyositis and dermatomyositis have been described in association with a variety of neoplasms, including lung, breast, and ovary carcinomas and lymphomas. Bohan and Peter (1975) point out that the claim that 71% of polymyositis found in men over 50 years old is a misquotation of the work of Shy and Silverstein (1965), mentioned above. Indeed, the muscular disorder considered by Shy and Silverstein (1965) is a late neuromyopathy, which is clinically different from polymyositis and dermatomyositis. The incidence of malignant tumors in patients with polymyositis in various studies reviewed by Bohan and Peter (1975) ranges from 15 to more than 30%. As for many forms of carcinomatous neuropathies, several factors (mainly, the interest in this type of association) may have distorted the figures reported in the literature. Regarding many types of carcinomatous neuropathies, we must conclude, as did Bohan and Peter, that adequate statistics are not available to confirm or deny an association between malignancy and polymyositis. Perhaps the association between neoplasia and dermatomyositis is more convincing.

CARCINOID SYNDROME MYOPATHY

Carcinoid Syndrome

More than 90% of the carcinoid tumors arise from the intestine argentaffin cells and are located in the region of the ileocecal valve. Occasionally, carcinoid tumors arise in the ovary, testis, or lung. They release active substances, such as serotonin, histamine, or kallikrein. These products (especially serotonin) are metabolized (inactivated) in the liver. Therefore, the carcinoid syndrome is seen only in patients in whom substances released by the tumor can reach the systemic circulation. This occurs when digestive carcinoid tumors produce liver metastases or when they arise outside the digestive tract. In these patients, serum serotonin and urinary 5-hydroxyindoleacetic acid may be markedly increased.

General symptoms of the carcinoid syndrome include acute reddish flush, which starts in the face and neck and is precipitated by emotional stress, periorbital edema, hypotension, tachycardia, abdominal pain, diarrhea, and asthmatic wheezing.

Carcinoid Myopathy

Muscle lesions observed in patients with carcinoid syndrome produce a progressive, marked proximal weakness. The affected muscles are mildly wasted and may be slightly tender to palpation. Cyproheptadine (Periactin®), a potent serotonin and histamine antagonist, improves the clinical manifestation of the carcinoid syndrome, including muscle weakness. Pathologically, atrophy and necrosis involve predominantly type II fibers. Central nuclei are present in both small (atrophied) and large fibers. There is no inflammatory reaction.

Relationship with Cancer and Pathogenesis

Carcinoid myopathy is very rare; only a few cases have been reported (Green et al., 1964; Berry et al., 1974; Swash et al., 1975). Nevertheless, it may result from a specific remote effect of cancer on the muscular tissue. Indeed, muscle weakness may be induced in rats by serotonin, and the syndrome may be prevented by antiserotonin drugs if they are given prior to serotonin administration (Patten et al., 1974). Other nonspecific factors, such as malnutrition caused by intestinal dysfunction, may contribute to muscle lesions in patients with carcinoid syndrome.

CONCLUSION

The so-called carcinomatous neuropathies account for a small percentage of neurological diseases found in patients with cancer. Their diagnosis should be considered only if all other causes of neurological lesions have been ruled out. The pathogenesis of these diseases is probably complex.

Certain metabolic encephalopathies, serotonin myopathy, probably Eaton-Lambert syndrome, and possibly osteosclerotic myeloma polyneuropathy result from a remote and specific effect of the tumor on nervous or muscle tissues. They may be considered as truly paraneoplastic phenomena.

Pathological examinations suggest that diffuse polioencephalomyelitis and sensory neuropathy, which are frequently associated, are attributable to a viral infection. However, this etiology has not yet been established.

The pathogenesis of all other forms of carcinomatous neuropathies remains obscure. Their relationship with the underlying malignancy is based on an alleged high incidence of these neurological disorders in patients with cancer. However, most reports of the incidence of this association are seriously biased by the interest generated by the association of cancer with unexplained neuropathies. The fact that most carcinomatous neuropathies do not respond to an adequate treatment of the tumor is a strong argument against a direct and specific remote effect of cancer on the nervous system.

REFERENCES

Allesi, D. (1940): Lesioni parenchimatose del cervellets da carcinoma uterino. *Riv. Patol. Nerv. Ment.,* 55:148–150.

Berry, E. M., Maunder, C., and Wilson, M. (1974): Carcinoid myopathy and treatment with cyproheptadine (Periactin). *Gut,* 15:34–38.

Bohan, A., and Peter, J. B. (1975): Polymyositis and dermatomyositis. *N. Engl. J. Med.,* 293:344–347; 403–407.

Brain, W. R., and Adams, R. D. (1965): Epilogue: A guide to the classification and investigation of neuromuscular disorders with cancer. In: *The Remote Effects of Cancer on the Nervous System,* edited by L. Brain and F. H. Harris, p. 216–221. Grune & Stratton, New York.

Brain, L., Croft, P. B., and Wilkinson, M. (1965): Motor neurone disease as a manifestation of neoplasm. *Brain,* 88:479–500.

Brain, L., and Wilkinson, M. (1965*a*): Subacute cerebellar degeneration associated with neoplasms. *Brain,* 88:465–478.

Brain, L., and Wilkinson, M. (1965*b*): Subacute cerebellar degeneration in patients with carcinoma. In: *The Remote Effect of Cancer on the Nervous System,* edited by L. Brain and F. H. Norris, pp. 17–23. Grune & Stratton, New York.

Case Records of Massachusetts General Hospital (1972): *N. Engl. J. Med.,* 287:138–814.

Case Records of Massachusetts General Hospital (1970): *N. Engl. J. Med.,* 283:805–143.

Case Records of Massachusetts General Hospital (1976): *N. Engl. J. Med.,* 294:1447–1454.

Case Records of Massachusetts General Hospital (1977): *N. Engl. J. Med.,* 296:1399–1405.

Cogan, D. G. (1954): Ocular dysmetria; flutter-like oscillation of the eyes and opsoclonus. *Arch. Ophthalmol.,* 51:318–335.

Croft, P. B., Henson, R. A., Urich, H., and Wilkinson, P. C. (1965): Sensory neuropathy with bronchial carcinoma. A study of four cases showing serological abnormalities. *Brain,* 88:501–514.

Croft, P. B., and Wilkinson, M. (1965): The incidence of carcinomatous neuropathy in patients with various types of carcinomas. *Brain,* 88:427–434.

Davis, L. E., and Drachmman, D. B. (1972): Myeloma neuropathy. *Arch. Neurol.,* 37:507–511.

Denny-Brown, D. (1948): Primary sensory neuropathy with changes associated with carcinoma. *J. Neurol. Neurosurg. Psychiatry,* 11:73–87.

Dorfman, L. J., and Forno, L. S. (1972): Paraneoplastic encephalomyelitis. *Acta Neurol. Scand.,* 48:556–574.

Ellenberger, C., Campa, J. F., and Netsky, M. G. (1968): Opsoclonus and parenchymatous degeneration of the cerebellum. *Neurology (Minneap.),* 18:1041–1046.

Fukumara, N., Takamori, M., Gutmann, L., and Chou, S. M. (1972): Eaton-Lambert syndrome ultrastructural study of the motor and plates. *Arch. Neurol.,* 27:67–78.

Green, D., Joynt, R. J., and Van Allen, M. W. (1964): Neuromyopathy associated with a malignant carcinoid tumor. A case report. *Arch. Intern. Med.,* 114:494–496.

Hildebrand, J., and Coers, C. (1967): The neuromuscular function in patients with malignant tumors. *Brain,* 90:67–82.

Ishikawa, K., Engelhardt, J. K., Fujisawa, T., Okamoto, T., and Katsuki, H. (1977): A neuromuscular transmission block produced by a cancer tissue extract derived from a patient with the myasthenic syndrome. *Neurology (Minneap.),* 27:140–143.

Kaplan, A. M., and Itabashi, H. H. (1974): Encephalitis associated with carcinoma. *J. Neurol. Neurosurg. Psychiatry,* 37:1166–1176.

Klingon, G. H. (1965): The Guillain-Barré syndrome associated with cancer. *Cancer,* 18:157–163.

Lambert, E. H., and Rooke, E. D. (1965): Myasthenic state and lung cancer. In: *The Remote Effects of Cancer on the Nervous System,* edited by L. Brain and F. H. Norris, pp. 67–80. Grune & Stratton, New York.

Levi-Montalcini, R. (1952): Effects of mouse tumor transplantation on the nervous system. *Ann. NY Acad. Sci.,* 55:330–343.

Mancall, E. L., and Rosales, R. K. (1964): Necrotizing myelopathy associated with visceral carcinoma. *Brain,* 87:639–656.

Mangalik, A., and Veliath, A. J. (1971): Osteosclerotic myeloma and peripheral neuropathy. *Cancer,* 28:1040–1045.

Moe, P. G., and Nellhaus, G. (1970): Infantile polymyoclonia-opsoclonus syndrome and neural crest tumors. *Neurology (Minneap.),* 20:756–764.

Monseu, G., Vanderhaegen, J. J., Stenuit, J., and Jadot, J. (1971): Etude clinique et anatomique de deux cas de générescence cérébelleuse subaiguë. *Acta Neurol. Belg.,* 71:324–344.

Norris, F. H., and Engel, W. K. (1965): Carcinomatous amyotrophic lateral sclerosis. In: *The Remote Effect of Cancer on the Nervous System,* edited by L. Brain and F. H. Norris, pp. 24–34. Grune & Stratton, New York.

Norris, F. H., Izzo, A. J., and Garvey, P. H. (1965): Brief report. Tumor size and Lambert-Eaton syndrome. In: *The Remote Effect of Cancer on the Nervous System,* edited by L. Brain and F. H. Norris, pp. 81–82. Grune & Stratton, New York.

Patten, B. M., Oliver, K. L., and Engel, W. K. (1974): Serotonin induced muscle weakness. *Arch. Neurol.,* 31:347–349.

Powles, R. L., and Malpas, J. S. (1967): Guillain-Barré syndrome associated with chronic lymphatic leukemia. *Br. Med. J.,* 3:286–287.

Richter, R. B., and Moore, R. Y. (1968): Non-invasive central nervous system disease associated with lymphoid tumors. *J. Hopkins Med. J.,* 122:271–283.

Roberts, K. B., and Freeman, J. M. (1975): Cerebellar ataxia and "occult neuroblastoma" without opsoclonus. *Pediatrics,* 56:464–465.

Ross, A. T., and Zeman, W. (1967): Opsoclonus, occult carcinoma and chemical pathology in the dentate nuclei. *Arch. Neurol.,* 17:546–551.

Rowland, L. P. (1965): Discussion. In: *The Remote Effects of Cancer on the Nervous System,* edited by L. Brain and F. H. Norris, p. 400. Grune & Stratton, New York.

Schlaepfer, W. W. (1974): Axonal degeneration in the sural nerves of cancer patients. *Cancer,* 34:371–381.

Senelick, R. C., Bray, P. F., and Lahey, M. E. (1973): Neuroblastoma and myelome encephalopathy. Two cases and a review of the literature. *J. Pediatr. Surg.,* 8:623–632.

Shy, G. M., and Silverstein, I. (1965): A study of the effects upon the motor unit by remote malignancy. *Brain,* 88:515–528.

Smith, B. (1968): Skeletal-muscle necrosis associated with carcinoma. *J. Pathol.,* 97:207–210.

Solomon, G. E., and Chutorian, A. M. (1968): Opsoclonus and occult neuroblastoma. *N. Engl. J. Med.,* 279:475–477.

Swash, M. (1974): Acute fatal carcinomatous neuromyopathy. *Arch. Neurol.,* 30:324–326.

Swash, M., Fox, K. P., and Davidson. A. R. (1975): Carcinoid myopathy. *Arch. Neurol.,* 32:572–574.

Urich, H., and Wilkinson, M. (1970): Necrosis of muscle with carcinoma: Myositis or myopathy? *J. Neurol. Neurosurg. Psychiatry,* 33:398–407.

Victor, M., Adams, R. D., and Mancall, E. L. (1959): A restricted form of cerebellar degeneration occurring in alcoholic patients. *Arch. Neurol.* 1:577–579.

Waddell, W. R., Bradshaw, R. A., Goldstein, M. N., and Kirsch, W. M. (1972): Production of human nerve-growth factor in a patient with liposarcoma. *Lancet,* i:1365–1367.

Waldenström, J. C. (1976): Specific activities of immunoglobulin produced by monoclonal gammapathies. Maladies of derepression. *Eur. J. Cancer,* 12:413–418.

Wilkinson, P. C. (1964): Serological findings in carcinomatous neuromyopathy. *Lancet,* i:1301–1303.

Wilkinson, P. C., and Zeromski, J. (1965): Immunofluorescent detection of antibodies against neurones in sensory carcinomatous neuropathy. *Brain,* 88:529–538.

Wilner, E. C., and Brody, J. A. (1968): An evaluation of the remote effects of cancer on the nervous system. *Neurology (Minneap.).* 18:1120–1124.

SUBJECT INDEX

Subject Index

A

Abscess, of brain, 93, 96
Acetylcholine, in Eaton Lambert syndrome, 134-135
Acute myelopathy, carcinomatous myelopathy, 178
in epidural space metastases, 22
Adenine-Arabinoside (ara-A), in treatment of Herpes Zoster, 93
Amphotericine B
in treatment of *Aspergillus* infection, 96
in treatment of *Cryptococcus* infection, 95
Ampicillin, in treatment of Listeria meningitis, 94
Amyotrophic lateral sclerosis
as form of carcinomatous neuropathy, 130
after radiotherapy, 25
Angioma, intraspinal versus epidural metastases, 20
Angiography, in brain metastases, 7, 8
Anoxia, as cause of metabolic encephalopathy, 122
Antidiuretic hormone
as cause of metabolic encephalopathy, 122
in treatment with vincristine, 55
Aphasia, 73
Ara-C, in treatment of encephalopathy, 53
of overt ML, 40, 60

Aspergillus, as cause of brain abscess, 89, 96
Ataxia, 51, 57, 72, 97
in BCNU and opDDD treatment, 58
peripheral neuropathy, 64
in procarbazine treatment, 58

B

BCNU
as cause of optic neuritis, 31
in treatment of meningeal leukemia, 49, 58, 65
Bleeding, intracranial, 113
Brachial plexus lesions
differential diagnosis, 45
caused by metastases, 44, 45
caused by radiotherapy, 45
Brain metastases
angiography in, 7
aphasia in, 6
and brain abscesses, 5, 10-11
and cerebrovascular diseases, 2
complementary examinations in, 7
CSF in, 8
diabetes insipidus due to, 5
differential diagnosis of, 10
distribution of, in certain areas, 1
EEG changes in, 7
main sources of, 2
melanomas of, 1, 9
and metabolic encephalopathies, 122